THE GREAT PHYSICIAN'S

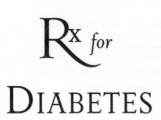

R^x *for*

DIABETES

JORDAN RUBIN

with Joseph Brasco, M.D.

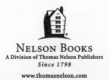

NELSON BOOKS
A Division of Thomas Nelson Publishers
Since 1798

www.thomasnelson.com

Every effort has been made to make this book as accurate as possible. The purpose of this book is to educate. It is a review of scientific evidence that is presented for information purposes. No individual should use the information in this book for self-diagnosis, treatment, or justification in accepting or declining any medical therapy for any health problems or diseases. No individual is discouraged from seeking professional medical advice and treatment, and this book is not supplying medical advice.

Any application of the information herein is at the reader's own discretion and risk. Therefore, any individual with a specific health problem or who is taking medications must first seek advice from his personal physician or health-care provider before starting a health and wellness program. The author and Thomas Nelson Publishers, Inc., shall have neither liability nor responsibility to any person or entity with respect to loss, damage, or injury caused or alleged to be caused directly or indirectly by the information contained in this book. We assume no responsibility for errors, inaccuracies, omissions, or any inconsistency herein.

In view of the complex, individual nature of health problems, this book, and the ideas, programs, procedures, and suggestions herein are not intended to replace the advice of trained medical professionals. All matters regarding one's health require medical supervision. A physician should be consulted prior to adopting any program or programs described in this book. The author and publisher disclaim any liability arising directly or indirectly from the use of this book.

Copyright © 2006 by Jordan Rubin

All rights reserved. No portion of this book may be reproduced, stored in a retrieval system, or transmitted in any form or by any means—electronic, mechanical, photocopy, recording, scanning, or other—except for brief quotations in critical reviews or articles, without the prior written permission of the publisher.

Published in Nashville, Tennessee, by Thomas Nelson, Inc.

Nelson Books titles may be purchased in bulk for educational, business, fund-raising, or sales promotional use. For information, please e-mail SpecialMarkets@ThomasNelson.com.

Scripture quotations are from the NEW KING JAMES VERSION®. Copyright © 1979, 1980, 1982 by Thomas Nelson, Inc. Used by permission. All rights reserved.

Library of Congress Cataloging-in-Publication Data [to come]

Rubin, Jordan.
      The Great Physician's Rx for diabetes / by Jordan Rubin with Joseph Brasco.
         p. cm.
      Includes bibliographical references (p.   ).
      ISBN 0-7852-1397-X (hardcover)
      1. Diabetes—Popular works. 2. Diabetes—Religious aspects—Christianity. 3. Diabetics—Rehabilitation—Popular works. I. Brasco, Joseph. II. Title.
   RC660.4.R84 2006
   616.4'6206—dc22   2005036830

Printed in the United States of America

1 2 3 4 5 6 QW 09 08 07 06

To my Great Grandpa Jacob and Great Grandma Leah, who suffered terribly and died from complications related to diabetes, and to the millions today who endure this painful condition. May this book offer you hope.

CONTENTS

INTRODUCTION

Time to Make a Change

In early 2004, Joey Hinson sat attentively while I spoke at a Wednesday night service at my home church, Christ Fellowship Church, in Palm Beach Gardens, Florida. That evening, I described how a thirty-nine-year-old acquaintance of mine had suddenly died from a heart attack, leaving behind a beautiful wife, four energetic kids, and a thriving ministry. "I had been asked to speak to this father and husband about getting on God's health plan, but we never connected in time," I said that evening. "How would his life—and those who mattered most to him—have changed if he had managed to turn around his health in time?"

A year later my church asked me to speak again, and this time Joey introduced himself after the service. "When you spoke a year ago, that story about that thirty-nine-year-old guy really did a number on me. You see, I'm also a husband and a father, and I felt like you were speaking directly to me. I knew I had to do something."

"Tell me about it," I said, intrigued, but humbled by what I had heard.

After he finished describing the events of the past year, I asked Joey if we could share his story with readers of *The Great Physician's Rx for Diabetes*. Here's what happened, in his words:

Throughout much of 2003, I began feeling horrible. This was something new for me because I thought I was in good shape, even for a guy who had turned fifty. I had played football in college—I lined up as an offensive lineman at Mars Hill College in North Carolina—so I was encouraged to "eat big" when I was growing up. It was hard to get away from that mentality after my college days were over, however. Over the years, I gained some weight—probably a good twenty or thirty pounds extra on my six-foot, two-inch frame. When I tipped the scales at 250 pounds a few years ago, I told myself to do something about it. I attended so many Weight Watchers meetings that I received a lifetime membership, but once I went off their food, the weight always came right back.

I think it's because I liked to eat southern foods too much. My weakness was fried chicken, black-eyed peas, and collard greens with the ham bone cooked in, or country-fried steaks dripping with gravy and yellow rice. Dessert had to be a rich chocolate cake or pecan pie.

Cheeseburgers and fries worked just fine for lunch. I worked as the transportation director at King's Academy, a private Christian school near my hometown of Royal Palm Beach, Florida, and a couple of times a week I borrowed the school's golf cart and drove to the Wendy's or Burger King located next door to school. People looked at me funny when they saw me ordering lunch from my golf cart, but I didn't mind. I was having fun.

What wasn't fun was experiencing a shortness of breath and lack of energy after turning fifty. Our house has a good-sized lawn that usually takes me several hours to mow. In the muggy Florida summer heat, I was too pooped to tackle the project. I'd lie down on the sofa, gasping for air, frightened by how fast my heart was beating. I felt really bad.

Donna, my wife, was naturally concerned, and I was bothered that I didn't have the energy to keep up with our youngest son, a ten-year-old. Then one Sunday night in August 2003, I was sitting in church, listening to the pastor, when beads of sweat formed on my forehead. My heart thumped like a bass drum, and I feared that a heart attack was imminent. "Lord, what should I do?" I prayed. Things got so scary that I thought about signaling for an usher to call 911, but I didn't want to create a scene in the middle of a church service.

I thought I was having high blood pressure problems since hypertension ran in the family. My symptoms calmed down a bit, so I toughed it out. I knew I should see a doctor, but I decided to wait a week or two for my annual physical. After my doctor poked and prodded around, he ordered tests on my blood and urine.

I'll never forget the phone call from the doctor's office informing me that I had type 2 diabetes.

Diabetes? That sounded serious. "Wait a minute," I said to the nurse. "I had my physical in the afternoon, so

I'm not sure if I fasted for my blood work. I want to get this checked again."

A repeat visit confirmed the test results. "I'm going to write you a prescription," my doctor said, handing me a slip and sending me on my way.

My prescription was for thirty milligrams of Actos daily to treat type 2 diabetes. As the months passed, however, I can't say that I was feeling better or that the medication helped me regain my energy. My concerns were raised by newspaper stories that Actos could cause liver damage.

Then I heard Jordan Rubin speak about the Great Physician's prescription for good health, and his message inspired me to make huge lifestyle changes in what I ate and how I lived. I asked Donna if we could buy our groceries at the health food store and purchase some of the whole food nutritional supplements that Jordan recommended. I think she fell over in shock because she had been encouraging me for years to live a healthier lifestyle.

I began eating a healthy diet filled with fruits, vegetables, and the right type of dairy, eggs, and meats. The days of ordering food at the Wendy's drive-thru lane in a golf court were long gone. Energy returned to the point that I could mow my big lawn again and keep up with the kids. Within a year, I had lost forty pounds and got down to my old high school playing weight.

When my annual physical came around in August 2004, I visited a new physician, but I did not disclose that I had been told a year earlier that I had diabetes. I wanted him to treat me with no preconceptions. So you can imagine my surprise when the test results from the lab confirmed that my cholesterol was good, my blood pressure was normal, and everything else was fine, meaning I didn't have diabetes.

Wow! Jordan Rubin was right. He said that if I followed the Great Physician's prescription, there would be a good chance that I'd reverse the damage I'd done to my body, and that's exactly what happened.

THE LATEST EPIDEMIC

Meeting people like Joey Hinson and hearing their stories are awesome, but my ears always perk up when someone says he has diabetes. You see, I had my own battle with diabetes back when I was a nineteen-year-old student at Florida State University a little more than a decade ago.

I chronicled my health odyssey in *The Great Physician's Rx for Health and Wellness*, where I described how my 185-pound body was attacked by Crohn's disease—a debilitating digestive order—along with a grab bag of other ailments: arthritis, chronic fatigue, hair loss, amebic dysentery, chronic candidiasis, prostate and bladder infections, as well as diabetes. Within a year I wasted away to 104 pounds and feared an early death.

Because I was fighting battles on so many medical fronts, I wasn't your typical diabetes patient, but I've never forgotten how both of my lower legs turned purple from extremely poor circulation. Now *that* got my attention. Although my doctors never suggested that I was a candidate for amputation, the thought of losing a leg crossed my young mind. If my health degenerated to a point where amputation was necessary, I really thought I would be better off dying.

Fortunately, and with great gratitude to my Lord and Savior, my health gradually improved, and the circulation in my legs returned to normal. Ever since I got well, I've carried a healthy respect for how diabetes impacts people's lives, and that impact is expected to double worldwide in the next twenty-five years. Researchers at the University of Edinburgh in Scotland are projecting a global rise in diabetes from 171 million in 2000 to 366 million in 2030. The greatest relative increases will occur in the Middle Eastern crescent, sub-Saharan Africa, and India, matching a similar rise in obesity rates.

Here in the United States, the alarm has already been sounded regarding diabetes. According to the most recent government statistics, around 18 million Americans—or 6.3 percent of the population—have been diagnosed with diabetes, and researchers estimate that there may be almost as many undiagnosed diabetics. The disease displays a strong ethnic bias based on its prevalence, in terms of percentage, among Native Americans, African-Americans, and Hispanics, as well as the aged.

Diabetes kills more than 200,000 Americans every year, ranking it as the sixth leading cause of death. Health authorities, however, believe that diabetes is underreported as a cause of death because many families and doctors, for one reason or another, choose not to enter the disease on the death certificate. A probable reason is that people often die of complications *relating* to diabetes—heart disease, strokes, high blood pressure, and kidney disease—so that disease becomes recorded as the cause of death.

Thus, many people are unaware that they even have diabetes. Although the affliction trails cancer and heart disease by considerable margins in the cause-of-death department, medical practitioners are calling diabetes a runaway epidemic because an estimated 41 million Americans have pre-diabetes, according to government estimates. Pre-diabetes is the period when people at high risk for developing full-blown diabetes demonstrate signs of intermittent elevated blood sugar levels. While their bodies are still capable of processing glucose—the energy that fuels the body's cells—their blood sugar levels are spiking like an aggressive teen driver running up the RPMs on his tachometer.

The "redline" image is apropos, especially since the American Diabetes Association has come out with red plastic wristbands as a way of creating awareness for the disease, just as cyclist Lance Armstrong introduced the canary yellow "Live Strong" wristbands as a fund-raiser for cancer research.

BACKGROUND ON DIABETES

Although millions of Americans and their families are affected by diabetes, I would venture to say that most people have a vague awareness of what diabetes entails. By definition, diabetes is a chronic degenerative disease caused by the body's inability to either produce enough insulin or properly use insulin, which is essential for the proper metabolism of blood sugar, also known as glucose. For those of you who last heard about insulin back in high school biology class, insulin is a hormone the body uses to convert sugar, starches, and other foods into energy for the cells.

To help you better understand the role of insulin, let me offer a short and simple description of how the body digests and absorbs food. The body's digestive process is considerably more complex than the following word picture, but this will give a general idea of how insulin is injected into the bloodstream.

When someone eats a meal, food travels from the mouth into the stomach before passing into the small intestines, much like the way food moves along various conveyor belts on *Unwrapped*, the Food Network program that shows viewers how their favorite foods are manufactured. Just as the featured item on *Unwrapped* is glazed, salted, roasted, or sugared as it wends its way through the factory, the food in the digestive tract is sprayed with various hormones, chemicals, and digestive juices. When food reaches the small intestines, it's bombarded with pancreatic juice containing pancreatic or digestive enzymes, which breaks the carbohydrates in the food down to the simplest form, glucose, which converts to blood sugar. When blood sugar levels rise, insulin is released to lower the blood sugar levels back to the normal range. The more carbohydrates you eat that are converted into blood sugar, the more your body releases insulin to lower that blood sugar.

Insulin accomplishes several tasks worth mentioning. The introduction of insulin stimulates the body to make fats out of other nutrients—proteins and especially carbohydrates—through a process known as lipogenesis. Why does the body do this? Because your body never wants to be caught short of gas in the tank. By storing the energy contained in sugar—or glucose—in fat cells, the body can call upon these "reserves" following physical exertion.

Unfortunately, with the lack of exercise in our couch-potato world these days, those reserves rarely get called on. Result: insulin levels spring out of whack after fat cells hang around too long. When blood sugar levels yo-yo for a long enough time, *diabetes mellitus* rears its ugly head in two forms: type 1 or type 2 diabetes. Doctors, however, are seeing increasing numbers of patients with double diabetes—symptoms of type 1 and type 2 diabetes.

Type 1, known as an insulin-dependent diabetes, means that the body does not produce enough insulin. To make up for the insulin deficit, the body must be supplied with steady amounts of insulin through a combination of controlled diet and daily injections of insulin, either extracted from the pancreases of cows or pigs or produced in laboratories in a synthetic form. In the last thirty years, medical scientists have discovered a way of manufacturing human insulin in bacteria and yeast, thanks to advancements in recombinant-DNA technology. Diabetics do not have to rely on insulin harvested from cows or pigs, whose supplies are being pinched by the limited number of animals set aside for this purpose.

Injections must be delivered with a needle because swallowing insulin is ineffective, the reason being that digestive juices in the mouth destroy insulin (which is a protein) before it reaches the bloodstream. My heart goes out to type 1 diabetics since it has to be incredibly painful and inconvenient to inject yourself in the thigh, arm, or abdomen every single day of your life. A new treatment protocol involves the use of an insulin pump, a small computerized device that delivers insulin into the body through a thin tube and needle inserted in the skin, usually somewhere around the beltline. I know several type 1 diabetics who are extremely thankful that their doctors switched them from injections to the pump, claiming that action has saved their lives.

Type 2 diabetes, a form of *non*-insulin-dependent diabetes (although some type 2 diabetics get so bad that they often require insulin), is difficult to diagnose and more challenging to treat. With type 2 diabetes, the pancreas does not produce enough insulin, or the cells ignore the insulin produced by the body. Since insulin regulates and maintains the body's circulation of sugar levels, the body's inability to metabolize blood sugar—for whatever reason—opens the door to a host of medical complications.

Insulin resistance by the body's cells may be caused by too much insulin production—a by-product of a high-sugar, high-starch diet. Insulin resistance can be compared to building up a callus while working a hoe in the backyard: when too much insulin is produced, the cells build up a defense, causing large amounts of sugar to remain in the blood. Often, the sugar in the blood reacts with the proteins to form advanced glycation end products, which hinder blood flow to the eyes, legs, and feet. Eating foods with antioxidants can stop their formation.

In addition to poor blood circulation, some of the common symptoms of type 2 diabetes include increased thirst, frequent urination, dry, itchy skin, poor wound healing, fatigue, bad breath, and irritability. The symptoms may sound vague, but in combination, these give a clearer indication of the onset of the disease. When full-blown diabetes is diagnosed—and the disease begins to take hold—additional physical problems and side effects become more stark: kidney failure, eye problems possibly leading to blindness, tooth and gum infections, and circulation blockages that cause heart disease or heart attacks. Some diabetic patients discover they have neurological problems and poor circulation, which manifest as tingly feelings in the hands or feet.

Diabetes is a leading cause of blindness, kidney failure, limb amputations, and heart disease. There's also a huge link between the rising rates of obesity in this country and the "epidemic" of type 2 diabetes. The fact that our government classifies two-thirds of Americans as overweight and 15 percent of children between the ages of six and nineteen as severely overweight does not bode well for the future of this country.

This is how serious type 2 diabetes is among the young: some demographers are worried that today's generation could be the first to live fewer years than today's life expectancy, which is 72.5 years for men and 78.9 years for women, according to the National Center for Health Statistics. Furthermore, researchers say that if present trends continue, one out of three children born after 2000 will develop type 2 diabetes, and those who develop type 2 diabetes before the age of fifteen will have a shortened life expectancy of approximately fifteen years.[1] That's sobering news, especially to someone who became a father for the first time in 2004.

CONVENTIONAL TREATMENTS

Diabetes is a serious disease that has no cure. The disease can be somewhat controlled, however, but that involves lifelong treatment and attention. Type 1 diabetics take daily insulin shots to maintain their blood sugar level within a normal or near normal range. Type 2 diabetics manage the disease through diet, exercise, and medication under the supervision of a physician.

Type 1 diabetics must monitor their blood sugar levels several times a day, incorporate thirty minutes of exercise into their daily activities, and spread their intake of carbohydrates throughout the day to prevent high blood sugar levels after meals. Insulin is the only medication used to treat diabetes directly, although some doctors prescribe medications like Cymbalta to treat depression or painful nerve damage in the hands or feet.

Type 2 medical treatments are more individualized. Doctors will focus on treatment plans that stabilize blood sugar levels, which revolve around eating the proper amount of carbohydrates each day. Since carbohydrates are the nutrients that most affect blood sugar, doctors will counsel their patients to "count carbs" so that they can maintain their blood sugar at a safe level. Registered dietitians are usually brought in to teach patients how to plan meals and count carbohydrates. Unfortunately, the current standard medical and dietetic recommendations are that diabetics substitute sugar and sugar-containing foods with artificial sweeteners and artificially sweetened products.

Doctors often recommend a low-fat, low-sodium diet with foods high in fiber to help balance blood sugar levels. Depending on their diagnosis, they may prescribe drugs that stimulate the pancreas to produce more insulin. Sulfa-containing compounds such as Glucotrol, DiaBeta, Micronase, or Prandin squeeze more insulin out of the body's cells. Other drugs help the body become more insulin sensitive: Avandamet, Rosiglitazone, and Metformin.

WHERE WE GO FROM HERE

From here on out, when I talk about diabetes, I will be referring to type 2 diabetes. My main reason is that more than 90 percent of diabetics are type 2, and the rapid increase in this form of the disease is prompting the alerts of an epidemic on the horizon. In addition, type 1 diabetes is thought to be largely an immune system disorder, and some in the medical world believe it's an auto-immune disease caused by a latent virus. More important, there is no proven way to prevent type 1 diabetes, but considerable evidence suggests that type 2 diabetes is highly preventable through eating right, living an overall healthy lifestyle, and embarking on an exercise program.

I believe even more can be done to prevent type 2 diabetes, and in the next seven chapters, I will be sharing the Great Physician's seven keys to health and wellness, which will give you and your loved ones the best possible chance to prevent diabetes or help you overcome diabetes by augmenting the medical treatment you're receiving.

My approach to diabetes is based on seven keys established in my foundational book, *The Great Physician's Rx for Health and Wellness:*

- Key #1: Eat to live.

- Key #2: Supplement your diet with whole food nutritionals, living nutrients, and superfoods.

- Key #3: Practice advanced hygiene.

- Key #4: Condition your body with exercise and body therapies.

- Key #5: Reduce toxins in your environment.

- Key #6: Avoid deadly emotions.

- Key #7: Live a life of prayer and purpose.

Each of these keys relates in some way to diabetes, as you will see. I believe each and every one of us has a God-given health potential that can be unlocked only with the right keys. I'm asking you to give the Bible's health plan a chance and incorporate these timeless principles into your life, allowing God to transform your health physically, mentally, emotionally, and spiritually.

No matter where you are in your health journey, I pray that God will meet you at your deepest point of need and deliver you from your health challenges.

Key # 1

Eat to Live

If you or a loved one has type 2 diabetes, you've probably noticed that friends and acquaintances who *don't* have this disease are often confused about your medical condition. They figure diabetes has something to do with sugar, but that's often the extent of their knowledge.

The general public harbors many misconceptions about diabetes. Some believe you're a prime candidate to develop diabetes if you're a closet chocoholic. This isn't exactly true; excessive consumption of sweets is more likely to give you a mouthful of cavities than cause diabetes. The body's inability to produce the right amount of insulin is the problem, not a secret love affair with Swiss chocolate. While everyone in the medical community agrees that sweets do raise blood glucose levels, people with diabetes can safely eat sugar. Diabetics shouldn't eat too much sugar, as I'll explain later in this chapter.

Others believe that diabetes can't be prevented. They say there's a strong hereditary link for those with a family history of diabetes, and if your parents have diabetes, then that's your destiny as well. While diabetes exhibits a strong hereditary component, "its rate of increase is too great to be a consequence of increased gene frequency," wrote Lyle MacWilliam in *LifeExtension* magazine. "Instead, evidence points toward the combined influences of lifestyle, dietary, and environmental factors."[1]

A generation ago, type 2 diabetes was unheard of among children, but the escalating numbers of youngsters with diabetes assert that the incidence of this childhood disease will become very serious over the next few decades. Experts are noting that type 2 diabetes is showing up with alarming regularity in heavy-set children who lead sedentary lives.

That's why I believe there's a link—medically and statistically—between the swelling ranks of diabetics and the other epidemic on everyone's lips—obesity. Not all overweight adults or children have diabetes, but it appears that nearly all type 2 diabetics are overweight. You need to look no further than a doctor's examination room for confirmation. Doctors on the front lines say that 99 percent of their patients with type 2 diabetes fit the preferred medical definition of overweight or obese, which is a body mass index (BMI) of 25 or 30 or more, respectively.

The body mass index is a mathematical formula that takes into account a person's height and weight and comes up with a corresponding number called the BMI. As a strict formula, the body mass index equals a person's weight in kilograms divided in height by meters squared. According to a body mass index table converted to pounds and inches for American use (these indexes are easily available online), the BMI breakdown goes like this:

- 18 or lower: underweight
- 19–24: normal
- 25–29: overweight
- 30–39: obese
- 40–54: extremely obese

As an example, someone standing five feet ten inches tall and weighing 167 pounds would have a BMI of 24—the limit defining one as having normal weight. Someone with the same height and weighing more than 209 pounds would have a BMI of 30, earning him or her a classification of obese on the body mass index scale. (Those who lift weights and have a large amount of lean body mass will be considered overweight or obese, according to the BMI scale. If you have a high BMI with a low percentage of body fat, you are not overweight or obese. This scale was created for the average nonathletic individual.)

If you find yourself on the upper end of the BMI scale, this would be an excellent time to ask your doctor about whether you should submit to diabetes testing, which usually involves a fasting blood glucose test or an oral glucose tolerance test. When the results come back from the lab, your doctor will inform you whether you have normal blood glucose, pre-diabetes, or diabetes. If the news is the latter, you will probably be counseled to lose some weight, undertake a regular exercise program, and reduce stress in your life—all ingredients of a major lifestyle change.

Losing weight is a *great* way to reduce the stranglehold that diabetes has on your body. A U.S. federally funded study called the Diabetes Prevention Program showed that losing between 5 percent and 7 percent of your body weight significantly reduces the risk of type 2 diabetes because a body carrying less weight uses insulin more effectively.

The Great Physician's Rx for Diabetes relies heavily on my first key, "Eat to live," which is an effective tool for losing weight. How does one eat to live? By doing two things:

1. Eat what God created for food.

2. Eat food in a form that is healthy for the body.

These principles involve eating foods and drinking liquids that give you an excellent chance of shedding pounds and maintaining the correct blood sugar levels. It doesn't mean exiting doughnut shops, fast-food restaurants, and supermarket checkout lines carrying bags of processed foods pumped up with sugars and artificial ingredients. Eating foods that God created in a form healthy for the body means choosing foods that allow you to beat back diseases like diabetes and put you on the road toward living a healthy, vibrant life.

For those with diabetes, this means consuming generous amounts of quality proteins, eating less high-glycemic carbohydrates such as grains, sugars, breads, pastas, rice, potatoes, and corn, and consuming more low-glycemic carbohydrates such as most vegetables and fruits, nuts, seeds, and legumes, and small amounts of whole grains.

When it comes to eating (1) foods that God created (2) in a form healthy for the body, I'm convinced that a diet based on consuming whole and natural foods fits within the bull's-eye of eating to live. Yet too many of the so-called foods sold in our nation's supermarkets were not created by God but were produced by employees in hairnets on an assembly line at some far-flung factory.

Like sheep following the next one off a cliff, we are filling our shopping carts with processed foods missing many of the nutrients that God intended us to receive and fortified with "modern" additives that rob us of health and vitality. As for eating out, don't get me started on how we've become a country that loves deep-fried, greasy food high in calories, high in fat, high in sugar, and—in most people's minds—high in taste.

Eating foods that God created in a form healthy for the body is an instant way to consume fewer calories. According to the Mayo Clinic, you consume only sixty calories when you eat one of these foods as a snack:

- one small apple
- one-half cup of grapes
- two plums
- two tablespoons of raisins
- one and one-half cups of strawberries
- two cups of shredded lettuces
- one-half cup of diced tomatoes
- two cups of spinach
- three-fourths cup of green beans

On the other hand, a Burger King Double Whopper with cheese comes out to a whopping 1,150 calories, or *twice* the amount of calories contained in *all* the fruits and vegetables I just listed!

I will be the first to agree that a diet of fruits and vegetables is too simplistic—and boring. Besides, a diet of low-cal fruits and vegetables does not provide the body with the full slate of nutrients that it needs, such as healthy proteins and fats. But let's get real: too many Americans are exiting fast-food restaurants, ice cream emporiums, and supermarket checkout lines with processed foods pumped up with calories like weight lifters on steroids. That's why we're having a nationwide problem with diabetes and obesity.

Contrary to popular opinion, there is no "diabetes diet." Foods healthy for everyone are foods that control blood glucose levels, but you must consume your foods carefully, especially carbohydrates. Every bite you take, whether it's a protein, fat, or carbohydrate, impacts your blood sugar and metabolism—and therefore your diabetes. Let's take a closer look at these macronutrients.

PROTEINS ARE PRACTICALLY PERFECT

Proteins, one of the basic components of nutrition, are the essential building blocks of the body. All proteins are combinations of twenty-two amino acids, which build body organs, muscles, and nerves, to name a few important duties. Among other things, proteins provide for the transport of nutrients, oxygen, and waste throughout the body and are required for the structure, function, and regulation of the body's cells, tissues, and organs.

Our bodies, however, cannot produce all twenty-two amino acids that we need to live a robust life. Scientists have discovered that eight essential amino acids are missing, meaning that they must come from other sources outside the body.

Since we need those eight amino acids badly, it just so happens that animal protein—chicken, beef, lamb, dairy, and eggs—is the only complete protein source providing the Big Eight amino acids.

The body needs the amino acids found in animal proteins, and the best and most healthy sources are organically raised cattle, sheep, goats, buffalo, and venison. Grass-fed meat is leaner and lower in calories than grain-fed beef. Organic and grass-fed beef is higher in heart-friendly omega-3 fatty acids and important vitamins like B_{12} and E, and is way better for you than assembly-line cuts of flank steak from hormone-injected cattle eating pesticide-sprayed feed laced with antibiotics. Eating protein supports weight loss and healthy blood sugar levels.

Fish with fins and scales caught from oceans and rivers are lean sources of protein and provide essential amino acids in abundance. Supermarkets are stocking these types of foods in greater quantities these days, and of course, they are found in natural food stores, fish markets, and specialty stores.

FAT OBSESSION

When I was a college student in the mid-1990s, I can remember sitting in the Florida State cafeteria and watching the coeds pick through their lunchtime salads while obsessing about the number of fat grams in the dressing. Low-fat diets were the craze back then, and anything with fat in it was Public Enemy No. 1. The thinking went along these lines, especially for the girls: *If you eat something with fat, then it will make you fat.*

As it turned out, consuming low-fat, reduced-fat, or fat-free foods didn't help anyone lose weight and may have actually caused metabolic problems. The problem with reduced-fat chips and fat-free yogurt was more than their poor taste: it turned out that these convenience foods had nearly the same amount of calories as the "full fat" versions. Since people thought they were eating low-fat, healthy food, they ate with abandon, which caused many to gain weight.

There's a compelling reason why low-fat foods were not the hoped for panacea. Chemically altered foods make things worse for the body, not better. God, in His infinite wisdom, created fats as a concentrated source of energy and source material for cell membranes and various hormones. Fats give foods flavor and aroma by adding creaminess, shine, smoothness, and moisture. In addition, fats are responsible for regenerating healthy tissues and maintaining ideal body composition, and they carry the fat-soluble vitamins A, D, E, and K throughout the body.

What types of fats in foods should diabetics eat? Ron Rosedale, M.D., author of *The Rosedale Diet* (Collins, 2004), believes that nuts, seeds, and nut and seed butters are great sources of fats that help buffer insulin (less insulin helps insulin sensitivity) and trigger the brain that the body is full.

People are often shocked to hear me say this, but this is why I say butter is better for you than margarine. Organically produced butter is loaded with healthy fats such as short-chain saturated fatty acids, which supply energy to the body and aid in the regeneration of the digestive tract. Margarine, on the other hand, is a man-made, congealed conglomeration of chemicals and hydrogenated liquid vegetable oils.

Fats and oils created by God, as you would expect, are fats you want to include in your diet. The top two on my list are extra virgin coconut and olive oils, which are beneficial to the body and aid metabolism. I urge you to cook with extra virgin coconut oil, which is a near miracle food that few people have ever heard of.

A Spoonful of Sugar

Of the different macronutrients—proteins, fats, and carbohydrates—carbohydrates have the biggest effect on blood sugar levels. Eating too many carbohydrates—especially those from refined sources—is a forerunner for diabetes because the body has a limited capacity to store excess carbohydrates. Too many carbs force the body to convert the excess carbohydrates into stored body fat.

By definition, carbohydrates are the sugars and starches contained in plant foods. Sugars and starches, like fats, are not bad for you, but the problem for those fighting diabetes is that the standard American diet includes way too many foods containing these carbohydrates. People with diabetes are usually careful about their intake of sugar, but you should be aware that sugar does not raise blood sugar levels any differently than similar amounts of calories from the starches found in many foods.

Still, health-care providers rightfully recommend that you avoid eating sugar unnecessarily, but that is easier said than done. Sugar and its sweet relatives—high fructose corn syrup, sucrose, molasses, and maple syrup—are among the first ingredients listed in staples such as cereals, breads, buns, pastries, doughnuts, cookies, ketchup, and ice cream.

Many people unwittingly eat sugar with every meal: breakfast cereals are frosted with sugar, break time is soda or coffee mixed with sugar and a Danish, lunch has its cookies and treats, and dinner could be sweet-and-sour ribs topped off with a sugary dessert. All those sweets can turn your health sour! A U.S. Department of Agriculture study in 2000 revealed that we eat an average of *thirty-two teaspoons* of sugar daily.

Many drink their sugar in the form of Cokes, Pepsis, 7-Ups, and Mountain Dews. Teen boys chug an average of three twelve-ounce cans of soft drinks daily, which contain forty grams of sugar in each drink. Teen girls are just behind at two cans a day,[2] which does not bode well for those with pre-diabetes or undiagnosed diabetes. A Harvard University study demonstrated that drinking more than one sugar-sweetened soft drink a day appears to significantly increase a woman's chances of developing diabetes. The greater risk comes from soda's excess calories and large amount of rapidly absorbable sugars, which send blood glucose levels soaring off the chart.[3]

The Great Physician's Rx for Diabetes calls for eating healthy proteins, healthy fats, and lower amounts of carbohydrates (sugars and starches). The combinations of foods you eat are important as well. I do not recommend that you eat fruit on its own because of its high sugar content; fruit should be consumed with fats and proteins, which will slow down the absorption of sugar.

STARCHY CARBS

Let's turn our attention to the starch side of carbohydrates. When carbohydrates are eaten, the digestive tract breaks down the long chains of starches into single sugars, mainly glucose, which is a source of immediate energy. As mentioned earlier, if these calories are not expended through physical effort, the body converts them to fat, and therein lies a weighty problem. As a culture, we are a little taller but a lot heavier than we were a generation ago; today we weigh twenty-five pounds more than our grandparents or parents did in the 1960s, with the biggest weight gains attached to men forty and older.

A trio of low-carb weight-loss plans—Atkins, South Beach, and Zone—have been flying off the shelf for years, with the *Atkins New Diet Revolution* spending an incredible six years on the *New York Times* bestseller's list. The main premise behind low-carb diets is that reducing the intake of carbohydrates like bread, pasta, and rice reduces insulin levels and causes your body to burn excess body fat for fuel.

My biggest beef with low-carb diets is that most of these health plans advocate a high consumption of meat products that God calls unclean (as I'll explain shortly), allow only limited amounts of nutrient-rich fruits and vegetables, and encourage the consumption of artificial sweeteners and preservatives.

Those with diabetes lean heavily on artificial sweeteners like aspartame-based NutraSweet or Equal, saccharin-based Sweet 'N Low, and chlorinated sucrose-based Splenda. Regarding Splenda, the chemical process to turn sugar into sucralose alters the chemical composition of sugar so much that it is converted into a fructo-galactose molecule. This type of sugar does not occur in nature, which means your body does not possess the ability to properly metabolize it.[4] It's my view that any artificial sweeteners should be treated as toxic substances to the body; they are not the answer for diabetics looking to sweeten their iced tea.

A Better Road to Health

I believe in a lower carbohydrate approach to treating diabetes and losing weight. The carbohydrates you want to consume are low glycemic, high nutrient, and low sugar. These would be most high-fiber fruits, especially berries; vegetables; nuts; seeds; and legumes; plus a small amount of whole grain products, which are always better than refined carbohydrates that have been stripped of their vital fiber, vitamin, and mineral components.

Eating unrefined carbohydrate foods, on the other hand, introduces fiber-rich foods into your body. Fiber is the indigestible remnant of plant cells found in vegetables, fruits, whole grains, nuts, seeds, and beans. Fiber-rich foods take longer to break down and are partially indigestible, which means that as these foods work their way through the digestive tract, they absorb water and increase the elimination of waste matter from the large intestine.

Good sources of fiber are berries, fruits with edible skins (apples, pears, and grapes), citrus fruits, whole grains (quinoa, millet, amaranth, buckwheat, and brown rice), green peas, carrots, cucumbers, zucchini, tomatoes, and baked or boiled unpeeled potatoes. Green leafy vegetables such as spinach are also fiber rich. Eating foods high in fiber will immediately improve your blood sugar levels by slowing the absorption of sugars into your bloodstream.

Chewing your food well will also slow the absorption of sugars into your bloodstream. If people tease you about "inhaling" your food, then you're eating too fast. I recommend chewing each mouthful of food twenty-five to seventy-five times before swallowing. This advice may sound ridiculous, but I know that a conscious effort to chew food slowly ensures that plenty of digestive juices are added to the food as it begins to wind through the digestive tract, and that's important for diabetics.

THE IMPORTANCE OF HYDRATION

While you're taking your time to chew your food, be sure to drink plenty of water during *and* in between your meals. Water performs many vital tasks for the body: regulating the body temperature, carrying nutrients and oxygen to the cells, cushioning joints, protecting organs and tissue, and removing toxins. Water happens to be the perfect fluid replacement; only God could come up with a calorie-free and sugar-free substance that makes up 92 percent of your blood plasma and 50 percent of everything else in the body.

F. Batmanghelidj, M.D. and author of *You're Not Sick, You're Thirsty!*, contends that diabetes "seems to be the end result of water deficiency to the brain" because the brain depends on glucose— blood sugar—as a source of energy. If you don't drink enough water, the kidneys can't function properly either. When the body is properly hydrated, however, the kidneys function normally, and the liver converts stored fat into usable energy. In other words, the liver—acting like a traffic cop—will direct the body to tap into its fat reserves when you're eating leaner foods, consuming less calories, and exercising regularly. You can greatly accelerate the liver's ability to convert stored fat into usable energy by consuming an abundance of clean, healthy water.

The importance of staying well hydrated cannot be emphasized enough. Dr. Batmanghelidj believes that many diabetics confuse hunger and thirst, thinking they're hungry when actually they're dehydrated. You should be drinking, at a minimum, at least eight glasses of water each day, which will give the body's vital organs the fluids they need as well as put a damper on the hunger pangs coming from the pit of your stomach.

If you're overweight, downing a glass of water a half hour before lunch or dinner will act like a governor on an engine, taking the edge off your hunger pangs and preventing you from raiding the fridge or pillaging the pantry. "You will feel full and will eat only when food is needed," Dr. Batmanghelidj says. "The volume of food intake will decrease drastically. The type of cravings for food will also change. With sufficient water intake, we tend to crave proteins more than carbohydrates. If you think you are different and your body does not need eight to ten glasses of water each day, you are making a major mistake," he said.[5]

Sure, you'll go to the bathroom more often, but is that so bad? Drinking plenty of water is not only healthy for the body, but it's a key part of the Great Physician's Rx for Diabetes Battle

Plan (see page 73), so keep a water bottle close by and drink water before and during meals.

COFFEE BREAK

Speaking of something to drink, is this country's obsession with Starbucks coffee healthy? Many health experts disagree about whether consuming caffeinated beverages such as coffee or tea is a good idea, but I must point out that coffee and tea have been consumed for thousands of years by some of the world's healthiest people. Although I'm not a huge fan of coffee or a coffee drinker myself, I will say that fresh ground organic coffee flavored with organic cream and honey is fine when consumed in moderation, meaning one cup per day. Teas and herbal infusions (the latter beverage is made from herbs and spices, rather than the actual tea plant) are another story all together.

Infusions of herbs and spices such as teas have been a part of nearly every culture throughout history. In fact, consuming organic teas and herbal infusions several times per day can be one of the best things you can do for your health. Green and white teas, for example, provide the body with antioxidants such as polyphenols, which help reduce cellular damage and oxidative stress. Studies have identified the anticancer compounds in tea as well as compounds that help increase metabolism. Teas and herbal infusions can provide energy, enhance the immune system, improve the digestion, and even help you wind down after a long day.

As far as caffeine is concerned, I believe that teas' benefits are better delivered in teas containing caffeine. Since tea leaves naturally contain caffeine, the Creator obviously intended for us to consume tea in its most natural form. Obviously, if caffeine tends to keep you up at night, you should avoid consuming caffeinated teas in the late afternoon or in the evening. For an after-dinner treat, try consuming a caffeine-free herbal infusion containing relaxing herbs and spices to help you wind down and decompress.

My favorite tea blends contain combinations of tea (green, black, or white) with biblical herbs and spices such as grape, pomegranate, hyssop, olive, and fig leaves. Even though I've never thought of myself as a tea-drinking type, my wife, Nicki, and I enjoy these biblical tea blends with dinner.

You'll find in my Great Physician's Rx for Diabetes Battle Plan (see page 73) that I recommend a cup of hot tea and honey with breakfast, dinner, and snacks. I also advise consuming freshly made iced tea, as tea can be consumed hot or steeped and iced. Please note that while herbal tea provides many great health benefits, nothing can replace pure water for hydration. Although you can safely and healthfully consume two to four cups per day of tea and herbal infusions, you still need to drink at least six cups of pure water for all the good reasons I've described in this chapter.

IF YOU GET THE URGE TO CHEAT

Let's say you're invited to a Super Bowl party. Tables are piled high with tantalizing hors d'oeuvres, crispy finger foods, and tempting sweets. You indulge. You graze. You keep on eating.

You're cheating. Your blood sugar levels are spinning like a slot machine.

How can you minimize the damage? According to Richard and Rachael Heller, authors of *The Carbohydrate Addict's Diet* (Signet, 1993), if you're going to cheat, then get it over with in a one-hour time frame. The Hellers say that when the body has been deprived of insulin-releasing foods high in carbohydrates, the body makes an adjustment. In other words, when you eat during one sixty-minute time frame, the body can be triggered to produce only so much insulin. Continue to snack longer—like right into the second half of the big game—and the body releases a second phase of insulin. That's not good when you have diabetes.

The Hellers advise that when you know you will be put in a situation that may sabotage your desire to eat well and control your diabetes, you should make sure that you eat a healthy, low-carb breakfast and lunch loaded with healthy protein, fat, fruits, and vegetables. When you're at the event, set your clock for one hour, and eat to your heart's content. During that hour, I would strongly recommend that you avoid consuming the worst of the "Dirty Dozen" (see page 22); other than that, you can "release the hounds," but only for that one-hour period.

In addition to the urge to cheat, diabetics often have to deal with food cravings. An efficient way to dampen cravings is to eat foods that aid the body's production of serotonin, a neurotransmitter that gives you a feeling of well-being. Foods known to help the body produce serotonin are cottage cheese, milk, cheese, chicken, turkey, duck, and sesame seeds.

NUTRITION IN A BAR

In an effort to eat healthy and lose weight, many Americans have turned to consuming energy bars as a convenient meal replacement or an in-between snack. Doing this may sound like a good idea, but in reality, many energy bars are no healthier than a handful of Tootsie Rolls. In fact many energy bars contain harmful ingredients such as artificial sweeteners, chemicals, preservatives, and synthetic nutrients.

If you find it difficult to sit down to a home-cooked healthy breakfast every morning, or if you find yourself frequenting the vending machines during snack breaks, you can eat a healthy whole food bar as a meal replacement, healthy snack, or after-noon pick-me-up. In my quest for providing others with healthy alternatives, I've developed one of the finest organic whole food bars available today, containing recommended amounts of pro-tein, omega-3 fats, fiber, and probiotics, along with compounds known as beta-glucans from soluble oat fiber. If you find it dif-ficult to stay away from treats in the employee break room, then check out these whole food bars. (For more information, visit www.BiblicalHealthInstitute.com and click on the GPRx Resource Guide.)

THE TOP HEALING FOODS

We've discussed many healthy foods in this chapter so far, but the following foods are musts for your diet. In addition, keep this in mind when you sit down to eat: you should consume the protein, fats, and vegetables first before swallowing any fruit, sweeteners, or high-starch carbohydrates like potatoes, rice, grains, and bread. I know it's hard to resist fresh bread when it's presented in a nice restaurant, but you would be better off having a piece toward the end of your meal.

1. Wild-caught Fish

Fish caught in the wild are a richer source of omega-3 fats, protein, potassium, vitamins, and minerals than farm-raised fish, which are kept in cement ponds and fed a diet of food pellets. You can purchase fresh salmon and other wild-caught fish from your local fish market or health food store. Many other fish are healthy as well, including sardines, herring, mackerel, tuna, snapper, bass, and cod.

2. Cultured Dairy Products from Goats, Cows, and Sheep

Dairy products derived from goat's milk and sheep's milk can be healthier for some individuals than those from cows, although dairy products from organic or grass-fed cows can be excellent as well. Goat's milk is less allergenic because it does not contain the same complex proteins found in cow's milk.

I do not recommend drinking 2 percent or skim milk because removing the fat makes the milk less nutritious and less digestible, and it can cause allergies. Yes, whole milk has more calories, but this is not an area to cut corners. I've seen research suggesting that the mix of nutrients found in milk, such as calcium and protein, may improve the body's ability to burn fat, particularly around the midsection.

3. A Wide Selection of Fruits and Vegetables

Nutritionists have long known that fruits and vegetables are low in calories and high in fiber content. As mentioned earlier, eating plenty of fruits and vegetables—five servings a day are recommended—benefits those wanting to lose weight.

I've described how fruits and vegetables satisfy your hunger with fewer calories. You're going to save hundreds of calories a day by substituting sweets with just-as-sweet in-season fruits. Many fruits and vegetables are high in water, which provides volume in the pit of your stomach, not calories. Since these high-fiber foods take longer to digest, you feel full longer. It's kind of like having gastric bypass surgery without all the nasty side effects.

4. Soaked and Sprouted Seeds and Grains

Like fruits and vegetables, sprouted grains, seeds, nuts, and whole grains are high in fiber. *Whole grain* means the bran and germ are left on the grain during processing. *Soaked grains* retain their plant enzymes when they are not cooked. This process greatly helps digestion.

5. Cultured and Fermented Vegetables

Often greeted with upturned noses at the dinner table, fermented vegetables such as sauerkraut, pickled carrots, beets, or cucumbers are overlooked by those on a diet, even though they are some of the healthiest foods on the planet. Raw cultured or fermented vegetables supply the body with useful organisms known as probiotics, as well as many vitamins, including vitamin C.

If you've never put a fork on any of these foods before, I urge you to sample sauerkraut or pickled beets, which are readily available in health food stores.

6. Healthy Fats

Foods high in healthy fats, including olives, avocados, nuts and seeds and their butters, olive oil, flaxseed oil, coconut oil, and butter produced from healthy animals, can be wonderful allies in your quest for weight loss. Extra virgin coconut oil has been the recipient of some great press the last few years for its ability to help balance the thyroid, aid in metabolism, and assist with energy production. Some experts recommend that people with thyroid and weight troubles should consume as many as two to four tablespoons of coconut oil per day. Make sure to consume healthy fats with every meal to provide satiety and slow the absorption of sugar into the bloodstream, thereby keeping blood sugar and insulin levels at an even keel.

A balanced thyroid plays a vital role in your metabolism. Mary Shomon, author of *The Thyroid Diet* (Collins, 2004), says that certain foods high in tyrosine assist the body in the production of the thyroid hormone T3, which helps you utilize more oxygen and burn more calories. Foods high in tyrosine are cottage cheese, egg whites, safflower seeds, and meats such as turkey, antelope, quail, and buffalo.

7. Herbs and Spices

The use of herbs (rather than rich sauces on meats) and spices (rather than dressings, creams, or oil) is an excellent strategy for weight loss. I'm not talking about dousing your food in table salt, which is high in sodium, but employing strong flavors such as garlic, chili powder, cayenne, curry powder, rosemary, and tarragon to add taste to the foods you eat. A particularly beneficial culinary spice for improving diabetes is cinnamon because of its ability to reestablish insulin sensitivity, which is significantly decreased by diabetes.

A chemical in cinnamon, called methylhydroxy chalcone polymer (MHCP), has been shown to increase glucose metabolism of fat cells twentyfold, according to research findings from the Human Nutrition Research Center, a branch of the U.S. Department of Agriculture. Researchers at the Beltsville Human Nutrition Research Center in Maryland gave sixty people with type 2 diabetes various amounts of cinnamon every day for forty days, while those in a control group were handed placebos. People receiving half a teaspoon of cinnamon daily experienced a drop in blood sugar, fat, and cholesterol levels by as much as 30 percent.[6] Researchers believe that cinnamon may delay the onset of type 2 diabetes for those at risk.

Since cinnamon is proving to be a wonderful spice for blood sugar levels, I recommend that you sprinkle cinnamon on a piece of toast or in a smoothie or even mixed with cottage cheese, honey, and raisins every day. If you're diabetic, you should incorporate between a quarter teaspoon and one teaspoon into your daily diet.

THE DIRTY DOZEN

Whether you're diagnosed with diabetes or not, there are certain foods that should never find a way onto your plate or into your hands. Here are what I call the Dirty Dozen:

1. *Pork products.* In all of my books, I've consistently pointed out that pork—America's "other white meat"—should be avoided because pigs were called "unclean" in Leviticus and Exodus. God labeled certain animals, birds, and fish "unclean" because they are scavengers who feed off trash—or worse.

2. *Shellfish and fish without fins and scales, such as catfish, shark, and eel.* In the Old Testament, God called hard-shelled crustaceans such as lobsters, crabs, and clams unclean as well. Their flesh harbors known toxins that can contribute to poor health.

3. *Hydrogenated oils.* Margarine and shortening are taboo.

4. *Artificial sweeteners.* Diabetics who can't drink Pepsi or Coke straight up often turn to diet versions sweetened with aspartame, saccharin, and sucralose, to name a few. Yet these artificial sweeteners are made from chemicals, and their safety has sparked debate for decades.

5. *White flour.* One thing we've learned over the years: enriched white flour is not a diabetic's best friend.

6. *White sugar.* If you're looking for a culprit to blame for the diabetes epidemic, then look no further.

7. *Soft drinks.* Run, don't hide, from this liquefied sugar. A twelve-ounce Coke or Pepsi is the equivalent of eating nearly nine teaspoons of sugar.

8. *Pasteurized homogenized skim milk.* Like I said, whole organic milk is better, and goat's milk is best.

9. *Corn syrup.* This is another version of sugar and even more fattening.

10. *Hydrolyzed soy protein.* If you're wondering what in the world this is, hydrolyzed soy protein is found in imitation meat products. Stick to the real stuff.

11. *Artificial flavors and colors.* These are never good for you under the best of circumstances, and certainly not when you're trying to lose weight.

12. *Excessive alcohol.* Although studies point out the benefits of drinking small amounts of red wine for the heart (part of the "French paradox"), the fact remains that alcohol contains lots of calories. Overconsumption of alcohol has wrecked millions of families over the years.

EAT: WHAT FOODS ARE EXTRAORDINARY, AVERAGE, OR TROUBLE?

I've prepared a comprehensive list of foods that are ranked in descending order based on their health-giving qualities. Foods at the top of the list are healthier than those at the bottom. When eating, practice portion control. Put less food on your plate than you usually do and see what happens. A Pennsylvania State University study found that reducing serving size by 25 percent can help you consume up to 800 fewer calories per day without reducing satisfaction.[7]

The best foods to serve and eat are what I call extraordinary, which God created for us to eat and are in a form healthy for the body. If you are struggling with your blood sugar and weight, it is best to consume foods from the Extraordinary category more than 75 percent of the time.

Foods in the Average category should make up less then 50 percent of your daily diet. If you are struggling with your weight, it's best to limit consumption of average foods to less than 25 percent of your daily diet.

Foods in the Trouble category do not promote weight loss and should be consumed with extreme caution. If you are trying to lose weight, you should avoid these foods completely.

For a complete listing of Extraordinary, Average, and Trouble Foods, visit www.BiblicalHealthInstitute.com/EAT.

Foods in the Trouble category do not promote weight loss and should be consumed with extreme caution. If you are trying to lose weight, you should avoid these foods completely.

For a listing of Extraordinary, Average, and Trouble Foods, visit www.BiblicalHealthInstitute.com/EAT.

 THE GREAT PHYSICIAN'S Rx FOR DIABETES: EAT TO LIVE

- *Eat only foods God created.*

- *Eat foods in a form that is healthy for the body.*

- *At mealtime, consume protein, fat, and veggies before sweets or starchy carbohydrates.*

- *Practice portion control by putting 20 percent less on your plate.*

- *Drink six to eight or more glasses of pure water per day, and drink eight ounces of water whenever you feel hungry.*

- *When the food on your plate is half-eaten, take a deep breath and ask yourself if you're still hungry.*

- *Eat foods like whole oatmeal or whole food nutrition bars, which contain beta-glucans.*

- *Sprinkle between a quarter teaspoon and a teaspoon of cinnamon daily into your foods.*

Take Action

To learn how to incorporate the principles of eating to live into your daily regimen, please turn to page 73 for the Great Physician's Rx for Diabetes Battle Plan.

KEY #2

Supplement Your Diet with Whole Food Nutritionals, Living Nutrients, and Superfoods

I don't see how people with type 2 diabetes can optimize their health without using nutritional supplements. My reasoning goes like this: because the body breaks down food to gain energy and nutrients, most of those with type 2 diabetes have gunked up the works through poor diet, lack of exercise, and consumption of too many foods with sugar. While my first key, "Eat to live," is a solid punch against diabetes, supplementing your diet with whole food nutritionals, living nutrients, and superfoods can knock this disease out of the ring.

I speak from experience because I began taking whole food supplements, along with probiotics and enzymes, when I was at my sickest. Once I ingested the right supplements (I had previously taken hundreds of the wrong ones), I noticed an immediate improvement in my health problems, including the color of my legs, which were purple from the lack of blood circulation and nutrients in my blood. Since then, I have a Cal Ripken streak going: I've taken nutritional supplements *every day* for more than a decade. That's at least 3,650 consecutive days for those of you keeping score at home.

Let me tell you about an average day for me. Whenever I sit down for a meal, I discreetly reach for a silver case and pop it open. I pick out a few whole food living multivitamins and a couple of "live" probiotic and enzyme capsules, and I wash them down with a glass of water. Later on during the day, I ingest a green food/fiber blend supplement. My "chaser" is a heaping spoonful of one of my absolute favorite supplements—omega-3 cod-liver oil.

Some of you may be suppressing a gag reflex, but my reason for taking this wide array of nutritional supplements is not because I fail to eat healthy. My wife, Nicki, is a wonderful cook armed with dozens of fantastic recipes built around free-range or wild meats, organic vegetables, healthy oils, and fresh fruits.

Because I travel a great deal, there are times when I find myself in settings where I'm served meals that aren't the highest quality. I think it's a fair statement to say that the typical American diet strays from God's design with its glamorous array of mass-produced foods replete with empty calories, refined carbohydrates, and woefully inadequate nutrition. Taking whole food nutritional supplements covers my bases and offers a concentrated source of nutrients that plant foods don't always provide, mainly because of depletions in nutrient-barren soils.

Back in biblical times, foods coming from the fields contained many more vitamins, minerals, enzymes, and beneficial microorganisms than what's sold in supermarkets today. For the past half century or so, we've been sterilizing our soil with pesticides and herbicides, using synthetic fertilizers, and not letting our fields lay fallow every seven years as God commanded, which means our food—even what is organically grown—doesn't pack the same nutritional punch as it did for our forefathers.

From the outset, though, please know that I'm not one who believes type 2 diabetes can be turned around with a bottle of pills. After years of study in naturopathic medicine and nutrition, I understand better than most that dietary supplements are just what they say they are—supplements, not substitutes for an inadequate diet and unhealthy lifestyle.

Starting Your Day Off Right

When I talk to diabetics about supplementing their diets, I begin with multivitamins, and I have good news to report about them. In a double-blind study, middle-aged and elderly diabetics who took a multiple vitamin and mineral preparation for one year avoided respiratory and gastrointestinal infections by more than 80 percent, as compared to those diabetics given a placebo.[1] Dr. Thomas Barringer, director of research at Carolinas Medical Center in Charlotte, North Carolina, said that diabetes can leave people prone to infections because out-of-control blood sugar compromises the immune system and leads to minor deficiencies of certain minerals that are lost in excessive urination.

Multivitamins play a role in preventing diabetes because certain ingredients—chromium, vanadium, and magnesium—promote healthier blood sugar levels. Chromium and vanadium mimic insulin and help the body produce more of the hormone. As for magnesium, scientists believe that the mineral gives the pancreas the nutrients it needs to produce insulin. The study of chromium, vanadium, and magnesium and their relationship to diabetes is not fully understood, but scientists are confident that this trio of nutrients can improve diabetes control.

While researchers continue their work, I'm confident that those with diabetes will greatly benefit from taking a quality whole food multivitamin that supplies highly bioavailable nutrients in proper balance. Multivitamin supplements are especially important to overweight diabetics because many obese individuals are nutritionally deficient, and the stress from dealing with diabetes day in and day out can deplete the body of certain nutrients.

The American Diabetes Association, on its Web site, referred to a study performed at Shaheed Beheshti University of Medical Sciences in Tehran, Iran, of all places. The researchers divided the type 2 diabetes study members into four groups:

1. One group was given zinc sulfate and magnesium oxide.

2. One group received vitamin C and vitamin E.

3. One group received all four vitamins and minerals: zinc sulfate, magnesium oxide, vitamin C, and vitamin E.

4. One group received a placebo each day.

After three months it turned out that the group taking all *four* vitamins and minerals (zinc sulfate, magnesium oxide, vitamin C, and vitamin E) experienced the greatest reduction in blood pressure, which eased some of their symptoms for diabetes.

A good whole food multivitamin contains many more ingredients than zinc, magnesium, vitamin C, and vitamin E. These types of vitamins contain different compounds such as organic acids, antioxidants, and key nutrients, which are all essential to good health. They are more costly to produce since the ingredients—fruits, vegetables, sea vegetables, seeds, spices, vitamins and minerals, and so on—are put through a fermentation process similar to the digestive process of the body, but they are well worth the extra money.

The *best* multivitamins are produced from raw materials by adding vitamins and minerals to a living probiotic culture. If you're scratching your head and saying, "Huh?" let me explain. Multivitamins are produced several different ways. Some are derived from vegetable, mineral, or animal sources such as cod-liver oil, wheat germ oil, or yeast. Other multivitamins are derived from processing that extracts vitamins from fish liver oil, soybeans, and other natural sources.

The most common form of multivitamins, however, is synthetically produced in a chemist's lab and is also the cheapest to produce. If you see ingredients such as sucrose, cornstarch, thiamine mononitrate, pyridoxine hydrochloride, ascorbic acid, or sodium metasilicate listed, your multivitamin is produced from synthetic materials. Synthetic multivitamins are never going to be as good or potent as ones produced from natural sources; studies show that synthetically made vitamins are 50 to 70 percent less biologically active than vitamins created from natural sources. Another giveaway is seeing the letters *dl* in front of the name of an ingredient. An ingredient named dl-alpha tocopheryl, for example, informs you that you're taking a synthetic version of vitamin E.

If you're currently on medication for diabetes, research suggests that you may be deficient in folic acid and vitamin B_{12}, which should be contained in your whole food nutritional supplements. Besides giving you nutrients in good balance, a quality whole food multivitamin contains certain minerals—chromium, magnesium, and vanadium—that help to balance blood sugar levels, which improves metabolism.

Whole food multivitamins also cover your bases because our food isn't as nutritious as it used to be because of soil depletion. These multivitamins come packaged in different varieties: tablets and capsules are the most common; powders and liquids are less widespread. I prefer caplets as a good delivery system to ensure the nutrients get where they need to go.

Open Up to Cod-Liver Oil

Those with type 2 diabetes not only have high levels of fat in their blood, but they also travel through life with low levels of HDL, the "good" cholesterol. Doctors in Denmark discovered that sipping spoonfuls of fish liver oil daily helps those with type 2 diabetes slash the high levels of fat—known as triglycerides—in their blood cells. I must point out, however, that results of eighteen trials over a ten-year period show that while fish oil lowers triglycerides, the supplement appears to have no statistically significant effect on glycemic (blood sugar) control.[2]

The best type of fish oil to add to your daily nutritional regime is omega-3 cod liver oil extracted from cod taken from the freezing waters of the North Atlantic. Cod-liver oil is one of the best sources for omega-3 fatty acids known to man—an extraordinary nutritional resource that has been acknowledged to play a leading role in the development of the brain, the rods and cones of the retina of the eye, the lubrication of the joints, and the body's inflammatory response. Omega-3 fatty acids are beneficial to those suffering from diabetes and obesity. Besides decreasing cholesterol and triglyceride levels, omega-3 fatty acids lower blood pressure and appear to have antidepressant and mood-stabilizing effects.

The golden oils extracted from the filleted livers of Icelandic cod may be an acquired taste, but after a decade of sipping spoonfuls of cod-liver oil, I'm at the point where I can drink the stuff right out of the bottle. If you can't "stomach" the thought of sipping omega-3 cod-liver oil, you can now take this important nutrient in easy-to-swallow liquid capsules. (For recommended products, visit www.BiblicalHealthInstitute.com and click on the GPRx Resource Guide.)

GREEN FOODS

I would hazard a guess that if you have diabetes, then you're not a big vegetable eater—especially the green leafy kind. If you're having trouble motivating yourself to eat your veggies, I know a way your body can receive more green foods, which contain nutrients not found in the typical low-carbohydrate diet. I recommend the consumption of green superfood powders and caplets. All you do is mix the powder in water or your favorite juice, or swallow a handful of caplets.

A good green food supplement is a certified organic blend of dried green vegetables, fermented vegetables, sea vegetables, microalgaes such as spirulina and chlorella, and sprouted grains and seeds. When you drink or swallow green foods, your body is taking in one of the most nutrient-dense foods on this green earth—but containing less than one-twentieth the calories of a Big Mac value meal.

This is what I call a real two-fer: not only is a green food supplement high in nutrients and low in calories, but it gives you the dietary benefits of whole food living nutrients, including improving digestion and elimination.

WHOLE FOOD FIBER BLEND

As mentioned in Key #1, fiber can be a diabetic's best friend. Consuming adequate fiber will ensure a feeling of satiety since fiber delays the absorption of sugars in the body and provides a sense of fullness. An additional benefit is that fiber improves regularity, which helps to efficiently eliminate toxins from the body. Since most of us get about one-fifth of the optimal amount of fiber in our daily diet, I recommend taking a whole food fiber supplement. Look for one that supplies your body with a highly usable, vegetarian source of dietary fiber.

When searching for a fiber product that's right for you, choose a brand made from organic seeds, grains, and legumes that are fermented or sprouted for ease of digestion. One of the preferred ways to consume whole food fiber is to take a combination green superfood/fiber blend first thing in the morning and just before bed—mix it with your favorite juice or water. When you do, you're giving your body more nutrition than most people get in a week while promoting maintenance of healthy blood sugar levels. (For a list of recommended whole food fiber products, visit www.BiblicalHealthInstitute.com and click on the GPRx Resource Guide.)

PROBIOTICS

By definition, probiotics are living, direct-fed microbials, or DFMs, which promote the growth of beneficial or "friendly" bacteria in the intestinal tract. Many diabetic people have digestive problems because they put around-the-clock pressure on the gut to digest everything coming its way, or they eat the *wrong* foods, such as unclean meats drizzled with rich sauces, processed snack foods, or icky-sweet desserts.

When I was attending Florida State University, I was sicker than a Georgia bulldog for a host of intestinal ailments, including the runs. After I introduced whole food probiotics into my system, my health improved immensely. What happens is that the probiotics crowd out disease-causing bacteria, viruses, and yeasts. If you're experiencing constant intestinal pain, then supplement your diet with probiotics. The most effective probiotics contain soil-based organisms (SBOs), multiple strains of lactobacillus and bifidobacteria, and the friendly yeast saccharomyces boulardii. (For recommended brands, visit www.BiblicalHealthInstitute.com and click on the GPRx Resource Guide.)

ENZYMES

When you eat raw foods such as salad and fruits, you consume the enzymes they contain. When you eat cooked or processed meals, such as those from a restaurant kitchen, however, the body's pancreas must produce the enzymes necessary to digest them. The constant demand for enzymes strains the pancreas, which must kick in more enzymes to keep up with the demand. Without the proper levels of enzymes from foods—either raw or fermented—or from supplements, you are susceptible to excessive gas and bloating, diarrhea, constipation, heartburn, and low energy. Do these symptoms sound familiar?

Digestive enzymes are complex proteins involved in the digestive process. They are the body's day laborers, the ones responsible for synthesizing, delivering, and eliminating the unbelievable number of ingredients and chemicals that your body uses during your waking hours. When your body produces enzymes, their job is to stimulate chemical changes in the foods passing through the gut. The pancreas, which takes a lead role in producing digestive enzymes for the body, has to keep up by producing pancreatic enzymes. Those with pancreatic problems such as cystic fibrosis usually require some form of digestive enzyme, but junk food diets, fast chewing, and eating on the run contribute to the body's inability to produce adequate enzyme production and the subsequent malabsorption of food. These problems get worse as we age, not better.

If you're seeking to minimize the consumption of high-enzyme foods such as bananas, avocados, seeds, and grapes—

which are high in sugars as well—then take plant-based digestive enzymes to ease the digestion of food. (You can find recommended brands by visiting www.BiblicalHealthInstitute.com and clicking on the GPRx Resource Guide.)

Protein Powder

Maintaining adequate protein levels is important for blood sugar control, which is why some diabetics drink protein powder shakes during the day. Careful, though: protein powders sold in warehouse clubs, drugstores, supermarkets, and even natural food stores are usually derived from soy, milk, or whey protein. These protein powders are highly processed and derived from cows injected with hormones and fed antibiotic grain. If you can decipher the ingredient list, you'll detect artificial sweeteners, flavorings, and additives. You have several healthier options: using a whey protein from grass-fed, free-range cows, a fermented soy protein, or a protein powder made from goat's milk.

Final Thought

There is no doubt in my mind that the right amount of high-quality whole food nutritional supplements will make a big difference in your diabetes. However, keep in mind that the term *supplement* means "in addition to," so I want to encourage you to base your health plan on eating healthy, organic food and using supplements such as whole food multivitamins, omega-3 cod-liver oil, green superfoods, whole food fiber, enzymes, probiotics, and high-quality protein powders to aid in your quest for a long and healthy life.

℞ THE GREAT PHYSICIAN'S Rx FOR DIABETES: SUPPLEMENT YOUR DIET

- *Take a whole food living multivitamin with each meal.*

- *Consume one to three teaspoons or three to nine capsules of omega-3 cod-liver oil per day.*

- *Take a whole food fiber/green food blend with beta-glucans from soluble oat fiber twice per day (morning and evening).*

- *Take an antioxidant/energy product with B vitamins, folic acid, and chromium with each meal.*

- *If you want improved digestion, take enzymes and probiotics.*

- *To ensure optimal protein intake, incorporate an easily digestible protein powder into your daily diet.*

Take Action

To learn how to incorporate the principles of supplementing your diet with whole food nutritionals, living nutrients, and superfoods into your daily regimen, please turn to page 73 for the Great Physician's Rx for Diabetes Battle Plan.

KEY #3

Practice Advanced Hygiene

All patients with diabetes must have a higher standard of hygiene if they are to control repeated infections and other immune system problems," wrote Kenneth Seaton, Ph.D., a pioneer in advanced hygiene and immune system regulation. Dr. Seaton, the author of *Life, Health, and Longevity* (Scientific Hygiene, 1994), believes improved hygiene—along with nutrition and exercise—are the principal ingredients for turning around the health of those with type 2 diabetes. Taking preventive measures against infections, especially during periods of high blood sugar, is very important.

I became aware of Dr. Seaton and his groundbreaking work when I was recuperating from my own serious health challenges. Dr. Seaton had discovered that ear, nose, and throat problems, which represent 80 percent of visits to doctors' offices, could be linked to how we touch our noses, eyes, mouths, and skin with dirty fingernails throughout the day. When we touch ourselves with our hands, we inoculate ourselves with germs that can enter the body through the mouth, a nasal passageway, or the corner of the eyes.

Dr. Seaton is an Australian microbiologist who lives with his family in the United States. He coined the phrase, "Germs don't fly; they hitchhike," after his studies powerfully demonstrated that germs were more likely to be spread by hand-to-hand contact as opposed to airborne exposure. If you want to remain in good health, keep the areas underneath the fingernails, around the membranes of the eyes, and in the front part of the nasal passageway as clean as possible. This information is particularly relevant to those with diabetes because your immune system may have been severely affected by the disease.

Those with diabetes may not be aware that the disease also weakens the mouth's germ-fighting abilities. High blood sugar levels worsen gum disease, and gum disease makes diabetes harder to control. Gum disease is estimated to happen three times more frequently in diabetic patients who have elevated blood sugar levels than those without diabetes.[1] The following are warning signs to look for:

- red, swollen, or tender gums, especially after brushing or flossing your teeth
- gums that have pulled away from the teeth, exposing part of the tooth's root
- oozing pus when you press on the gums (although it would seem hard not to notice this)
- loose teeth moving away from each other

Oral infections are another manifestation of diabetes. When clusters of germs cause problems in one area of your mouth, you should seek medical and dental attention.

But you can take steps to avoid reaching that point by practicing advanced hygiene.

A PRIMER ON GERMS

How do you get germs on your hands? By shaking hands with others or touching things they touched: handrails, doorknobs, shopping carts, paper money, coins, and food. Whenever you read about a breakout of E. coli infections, you can bet your last dollar that it can be traced to a restaurant where workers and cooks who were tossing salads and handling food didn't wash their hands after using the bathroom.

I know this stuff isn't pleasant dinnertime conversation, but hygiene is part of the Great Physician's prescription for health and wellness, which is why I've been following an advanced hygiene protocol for more than a decade with startling results in my life: no lingering head colds, no nagging sinus infections, and no acute respiratory illnesses to speak of for many years.

Here's what I do: each morning and evening, I dip both hands into a tub of semisoft soap and dig my fingernails into the cream. Then I work the special cream soap around the tips of my fingers, cuticles, and fingernails for fifteen to thirty seconds. When I'm finished, I lather my hands for fifteen seconds before rinsing them under running water. After my hands are clean, I take another dab of semisoft soap and wash my face.

My second step involves a procedure that I call a facial dip. I fill my washbasin or a clean, large bowl with warm but not hot water. When enough water is in the basin, I add one or two table-spoons of regular table salt and two eyedroppers of a mineral-based facial solution into the cloudy water. I mix everything with my hands, and then I bend over and dip my face into the cleansing matter, opening my eyes several times to allow the membranes to be cleaned. After coming up for air, I dunk my head a second time and blow bubbles through my nose. "Sink snorkeling," I call it.

My final two steps of advanced hygiene involve applying very diluted drops of hydrogen peroxide and minerals into my ears for thirty to sixty seconds to cleanse the ear canals, and brushing my teeth with an essential oil-based tooth solution to cleanse my mouth of unhealthy germs.

Following this advanced hygiene protocol involves discipline; you have to remind yourself to do it until it becomes an ingrained habit. I find it easier to follow these steps in the morning and before bed. Since starting my hygiene regimen, I just don't feel clean without it. And the best part is, it takes less than three minutes from start to finish.

I urge you to incorporate advanced hygiene into your life, paying special attention to washing your hands periodically, especially after you've been in public situations and shaken the hands of a few friends. I don't want to drive up anyone's paranoia meter, but sometimes our biggest exposure to germs all week happens after church, when we're shaking hands with old friends and new acquaintances in the foyer. All the while, we're exchanging a garden variety of bacteria, allergens, environmental toxins, and viruses from one part of the body to another. So wash those hands well—and often.

℞ THE GREAT PHYSICIAN'S Rx FOR DIABETES: PRACTICE ADVANCED HYGIENE

- *Wash your hands regularly, paying special attention to removing germs from underneath your fingernails.*

- *Cleanse your nasal passageways and the mucous membranes of the eyes daily by performing a facial dip.*

- *Cleanse the ear canals at least twice per week.*

- *Use an essential oil-based tooth solution daily to remove germs from the mouth and improve the health of the gums.*

Take Action

To learn how to incorporate the principles of practicing advanced hygiene into your daily regimen, please turn to page 73 for the Great Physician's Rx for Diabetes Battle Plan.

KEY #4

Condition Your Body with Exercise and Body Therapies

Ron Cook, a correctional officer who supervised seventy-five deputies at Sedgwick County Jail in Wichita, Kansas, liked to start the day by visiting Squeaky's Doughnuts next door to the county lockup.

I know there's a joke somewhere about a cop and a doughnut shop, but that was Ron's daily routine. He was partial to the buttermilk doughnuts with a sugar glaze, and he enjoyed eating two of them with his sugared coffee. Ron arrived at 5:30 every morning, giving him a chance to hang out with other sheriff's deputies before the start of their shift at 6:00 a.m.

Fifty years old now, Ron was recently forced into retirement because of his diabetic condition. Years of poor diet, lack of sleep, and no exercise had taken its toll on him and his personal life: he's been married four times. So when Ron heard me speak at Central Christian Church in Wichita, he was ready to make major lifestyle changes, including getting enough rest and starting an exercise program.

Getting enough sleep was always difficult for Ron, who carried the stress of running a correctional facility with 1,400 prisoners on his broad shoulders. Most nights, Ron didn't get more than five or six hours of shut-eye, leaving him feeling unrefreshed when the alarm clock jangled him awake at 4:45 a.m.

Ron was among the one hundred million Americans who get

up each morning without enough proper rest. The root causes of our national sleep debt are overcrowded schedules, the desire to accomplish one more thing before retiring, and too much stimulation from watching TV. This is a shame because those who sleep less than five hours are 2.5 times more likely to have diabetes, according to a study performed at Boston University.[1] Dr. Daniel Gottlieb, the study's coauthor, said researchers adjusted the statistics to remove any influence of gender, age, race, or body type. According to the study, a lack of rest impairs the body's ability to process glucose, a cause of diabetes. For type 2 diabetics struggling to lose weight, not enough sleep boosts the appetite, especially for high-calorie, high-carbohydrate foods.

Sleep is a major regulator of leptin, a hormone that tells the brain that it doesn't need more food, and ghrelin, a different hormone that triggers hunger. When test subjects slept only four hours nightly, leptin levels decreased by 18 percent, and ghrelin levels increased 28 percent.[2] Translation: they had the munchies for a midnight snack.

Dr. Gottlieb said his study bolstered the common recommendation for sleeping seven or eight hours a night, which I would amend to something closer to eight hours than to seven hours. Eight hours is the number to shoot for because when people can control the amount of time they sleep, such as in a sleep laboratory, they naturally sleep eight hours in a twenty-four-hour period.

Like millions of Americans, my wife, Nicki, and I wish we could catch eight wonderful, blissful hours of sleep, but as parents of an energetic toddler, we've gotten used to getting up in the middle of the night to tend to him. If Joshua is cooperative, we get our eight hours, although as Nicki would remind me, I'm speaking for myself since moms often sleep with one eye open and the other closed.

What I've found most beneficial is following the advice of my friend and colleague Dr. Joseph Mercola of Mercola.com, who told me that one hour of sleep *before* midnight is equal to four hours of sleep *after* midnight. I know Dr. Joe is right because when I go to bed really late, say around 2:00 a.m., I don't feel well in the morning—or the next day. But when I go to bed before midnight, I wake up refreshed and ready to hit the day.

THERE'S MORE THAN JUST SLEEP

Sleep is just one of a half-dozen body therapies that you should incorporate into your lifestyle. A close cousin to sleep is rest, which also seems to be in short supply these days. We don't get enough rest because of our "shop until you drop" culture that's available 24/7. In the last decade, neighborhood supermarkets have begun to stay open all night long, as have chain pharmacy stores. When the latest Harry Potter books go on sale, bookstores stay open in the middle of the night so they can officially begin selling them at midnight. And shopping online is perfect for someone trying to squeeze in one more purchase that day.

Busy weekends exacerbate the problem. Malls and other shopping emporiums vie for shoppers' dollars with alluring sales, and many families run themselves ragged driving their kids to all the soccer, T-ball, and lacrosse games. Woe to the parents with children good enough to play on travel teams.

Families need a time of rest by taking a break from the rat race on Saturday or Sunday. God created the earth and the heavens in six days and rested on the seventh, giving us an example and a reminder that we need to take a break from our labors. Just as triathletes and other high-performance athletes are careful to give their bodies one day off a week, we should be as well. Otherwise, we're prime candidates for burnout.

GIVE ME TWENTY OR DROP

A body therapy that is just as important to diabetes is exercise. Many who have diabetes are overweight and often obese, and exercise may be as foreign as a Roberto Benigni film. Exercise doeth a body good, whether you're an overweight diabetic or not.

You cannot afford *not* to exercise, and if that means scheduling an appointment with a trainer at a gym, then do so. Trying to control your blood sugar or lose weight without exercising would be like trying to ace a final exam without studying. While it can be done, ninety-nine times out of a hundred you can't lose weight—or at least sustain any weight loss—without stoking the body's furnace to burn up reserves of fat.

Exercise is also key to managing diabetes and blood glucose levels. When you huff and puff, the body demands extra energy (in the form of glucose) for the muscles, which lowers blood glucose levels. Moderate exercise prompts the muscles to ask for glucose at nearly twenty times the normal rate. In addition, when you exercise faithfully, you will

- improve your body's use of insulin.
- burn excess body fat, which results in improved insulin sensitivity.
- improve muscle strength and increase bone density.
- lower blood pressure levels and reduce the risk of heart disease.
- lower "bad" LDL cholesterol levels and increase "good" HDL cholesterol levels.

What kind of exercise should you do when you have diabetes? If the last time you darkened a gym was when George Herbert Walker Bush lived in the White House, I know a great way to get back into the exercise game. It's called *functional fitness,* and this form of gentle exercise will get your body burning calories and improve agility. The idea behind functional fitness is to train movements, not muscles, as you build up cardiovascular endurance and the body's core muscles. You do this through performing real-life activities in real-life positions. (Please visit www.GreatPhysiciansRx.com for in-depth instructions of functional fitness exercises.)

Functional fitness uses body weight exercises, but can also employ dumbbells, mini trampolines, and stability balls. It is gaining popularity around the country. Instructors at LA Fitness, Bally Total Fitness, and local YMCAs put you through a series of exercises that mimic everyday life. You're asked to perform squats with feet apart, feet together, and one back with the other forward. You're asked to do reaching lunges, push-ups against a wall, and "supermans" that involve lying on the floor and lifting up your right arm while lifting your left leg into a fully extended position. What you're *not* asked to perform are high-impact exercises like those found in energetic, pulsating aerobics classes.

A functional fitness program provides an entry-level approach to exercise, increases strength in the daily tasks of life, and when done twice a day for five to fifteen minutes at a time, burns calories so that you can lose unwanted weight.

One surefire way to improve your health is to start walking, which is an excellent form of exercise for those battling diabetes. Walking is a low-impact but surprisingly effective exercise that places a gentle strain on the heart muscle as you work up to better fitness.

Walking around the neighborhood or on a treadmill at a fitness facility can be done when it's most convenient for you. You can walk before work, during your lunch hour, or before dinner. You set the pace; you decide how much to put into this exercise.

If possible, you can kill two birds with one stone by walking in the sunlight. Exposing your face and skin to sunlight is another body therapy I recommend because it gives the body a chance to synthesize vitamin D from the ultraviolet rays of the sun. Getting some sun—whether on a walk or sitting in a chair outside work or in the backyard—has important health ramifications for those with diabetes. The vitamin D in sunlight, when synthesized by the body, augments the production of insulin. When not enough insulin is present in the bloodstream, the body naturally wants to raise insulin levels, and it does that by signaling a hunger for high-carbohydrate foods. Sun exposure will help your metabolism and insulin levels.

I recommend finding at least fifteen minutes of sunlight a day to capture the vitamin D in the rays of the sun. If you're living underneath a gray cloud cover, then take one-to-three teaspoons or three-to-nine capsules of omega-3 cod liver oil daily, which is another important source of vitamin D.

Hot and Cold Ideas

In *The Great Physician's Rx for Health and Wellness,* I devoted an entire section to hydrotherapy, aromatherapy, and music therapy. These forms of therapy encourage relaxation, reduce stress, and flush out toxins.

Hydrotherapy comes in the form of baths, showers, washing, and wraps—using hot *and* cold water. For instance, I wake up with a hot shower in the mornings, but then I turn off the hot water and stand under the brisk cold water for about a minute, which totally invigorates me. Cold water stimulates the body and boosts oxygen use in the cells, while hot water dilates blood vessels, which improves blood circulation (important for those with diabetic neuropathy) and transports more oxygen to the brain.

The next time you shower, warm up your body first with hot water. Then slowly turn off the hot water until the cool water becomes cold. Stay under the cold nozzle for at least a minute. You'll feel an increase in energy while improving body awareness.

Hot baths are good for those with diabetes because the hot water on skin expands blood vessels, filling them with blood. Taking a cold or cool shower afterward causes constriction, which improves blood flow. I recommend adding essential oils or herbs to the bath to enhance the therapeutic benefits.

Sitting in a sauna is another form of hydrotherapy. Some with diabetes do not have normal temperature sensation, particularly in their feet, so pay attention. A sauna will not make you lose weight, if that's what you're interested in. Sure, you'll sweat a lot, but any weight loss is likely to be a form of water loss from perspiration. You'll gain weight right back as soon you replace those lost fluids, but you will rid your body of toxins, and that's a good thing for anyone with diabetes.

My final two body therapies—aromatherapy and music therapy—elevate mood, which is certainly an issue when you're dealing with a serious disease like diabetes. In aromatherapy, essential oils from plants, flowers, and spices can be introduced to your skin and pores either by rubbing them in or by inhaling their aromas. The use of these essential oils will give you an emotional lift if you're struggling with your condition. Try rubbing a few drops of myrtle, coriander, hyssop, galbanum, or frankincense onto the palms, then cup your hands over your mouth and nose and inhale. A deep breath will invigorate the spirit.

So will listening to soft and soothing music that promotes relaxation and healing. I know what I like when it comes to music therapy: contemporary praise and worship music. No matter what works for you, you'll find that listening to uplifting "mood" music is healing.

R℞ THE GREAT PHYSICIAN'S Rx FOR DIABETES: CONDITION YOUR BODY WITH EXERCISE AND BODY THERAPIES

- Make a commitment and an appointment to exercise at least three times a week.

- Incorporate five to fifteen minutes of functional fitness into your daily schedule.

- Take a brisk walk and see how much better you feel at the end of the day.

- Go to sleep earlier, paying close attention to how much sleep you get before midnight. Do your best to get eight hours of sleep nightly. Remember that sleep is the most important nonnutrient you can incorporate to improve your health.

- End your next shower by changing the water temperature to cool (or cold) and standing underneath the spray for one minute.

- During your next break from work, sit outside in a chair and face the sun. Soak up the rays for ten or fifteen minutes.

- Incorporate essential oils into your daily life.

- Play worship music in your home, in your car, or on your iPod. Focus on God's plan for your life.

Take Action

To learn how to incorporate the principles of conditioning your body with exercise and body therapies into your daily regimen, please turn to page 73 for the Great Physician's Rx for Diabetes Battle Plan.

KEY #5

Reduce Toxins in Your Environment

In my last chapter, I introduced Ron Cook, a correctional officer from Wichita, Kansas. There's something more you should
know about Ron's story because it relates directly to the topic of
this chapter, which is reducing the amount of toxins in your
environment.

Ron told me that after reading an earlier book of mine,
Patient, Heal Thyself, he put two and two together: the reason why
his gut was so "messed up," as he described it, was from mercury
poisoning in his body, which would come from the foods he ate
and amalgam fillings in his teeth. When he adopted the principles
behind the *Great Physician's Rx for Health and Wellness,* however,
his blood sugar levels were cut in half. But check this out: one
time when he went swimming in a heavily chlorinated pool, his
blood sugar levels shot back up to their old levels again!

Stories like Ron's remind me that we all have toxins inside our
bodies because they are present everywhere in our environment—the air we breathe, the water we drink or swim in, the
lotions and cosmetics we rub on our skin, the products we use to
clean our homes, and even the toothpaste we dab on our tooth-
brushes. If your blood and urine were tested, lab technicians
would uncover dozens of toxins in your bloodstream, including
PCBs (polychlorinated biphenyls), dioxins, furans, trace metals,
phthalates, VOCs (volatile organic compounds), and chlorine.

Some toxins are water soluble, meaning they are rapidly passed out of the body and present little harm. Unfortunately many more toxins are fat soluble, meaning that it can take months or years before they are completely eliminated from your system. Some of the better known fat-soluble toxins are dioxins, phthalates, and chlorine, and when they are not eliminated from the body, they become stored in your fatty tissues. "Consider those love handles as a hiding place for stored toxins and poisons," says Don Colbert, M.D. and author of *Toxic Relief.* "In other words, fat is usually toxic, too."[1]

The best way to flush fat-soluble toxins out of your bloodstream is to increase your intake of drinking water (which I'll get into shortly) so that you will excrete toxins via the kidneys and urinary tract; consume a whole food fiber/green food blend to aid in the elimination of toxins from the bowel; increase perspiration through exercise and sauna baths to eliminate toxins through the lymphatic system; and practice deep breathing to eliminate toxins from the lungs. Dietary detoxification strategies include increasing the intake of high-enzyme raw fruits and vegetables, increasing dietary fiber, and eating leaner meats, especially grass-fed or pastured beef or bison and wild-caught fish. Remember: most commercially produced beef, chicken, and pork act as chemical magnets for toxins in the environment, so they will not be as healthy as eating grass-fed beef. In addition, consuming organic produce purchased at health food stores, roadside stands, and farmers' markets will expose you to less pesticide residues, as compared to conventionally grown fruits and vegetables.

Canned tuna, because of its high mercury levels, is another

food to be careful of, which is why I recommend no more than two cans of tuna per week. Due to environmental contamination, metallic particles of mercury, lead, and aluminum continue to be found in the fatty tissues of tuna, swordfish, and king mackerel. Shrimp and lobster, which are shellfish that scavenge the ocean floor, are unclean meats that should be eliminated from your diet.

WHAT TO DRINK

Every diet book on the shelf touts the health benefits of drinking water, and I second that advice. Water is especially important because of its ability to flush out toxins and other metabolic wastes from the body, and overweight people with diabetes tend to have larger metabolic loads.

Increasing your intake of water will speed up your metabolism—which can lead to weight loss—and allow your body to assimilate nutrients from the foods you eat and the nutritional supplements you take. Since water is the primary resource for carrying nutrients throughout the body, a lack of adequate hydration results in metabolic wastes accumulating in your body—a form of self-poisoning. That's why I preach that the importance of drinking enough water cannot be overstated: water is a life force involved in nearly every bodily process, from efficient digestion to healthy blood circulation.

Yet many with diabetes eschew water for a pale imitation—diet drinks, thinking that sodas like Diet Coke, Diet Dr. Pepper, and Diet Pepsi are okay to drink because they do not contain any sugar. I believe, however, that these diet drinks are just as bad or worse for diabetics than regular soda because they contain artificial sweeteners like aspartame, acesulfame K, or sucralose.

Even though the Food and Drug Administration has approved the use of artificial sweeteners in drinks (and foods), these chemical food additives may prove to be detrimental to your health in the long term. And if you're thinking that "energy drinks" like Red Bull and Sobe Adrenaline Rush are a solution to hydration, then let me remind you that these drinks come "fortified" with caffeine and unhealthy amino acids.

Nothing beats plain old water for those with diabetes, especially those who are obese. Diabetics should take note of what F. Batmanghelidj, M.D. and author of *You're Not Sick, You're Thirsty!*, says about the topic:

> Dry mouth is one of the very last indicators of dehydration of the body. By the time dry mouth becomes an indicator of water shortage, many delicate functions of the body have been shut down and prepared for depletion. A dehydrated body loses sophistication and versatility. One example is juvenile diabetes, in which the insulin-producing cells of the pancreas are sacrificed as a result of persistent dehydration.[2]

So for the second time in this book, I urge you to drink a lot of water. Cold or lukewarm, it doesn't matter. Water helps you digest your meals more efficiently, reduces fluid retention, and prevents constipation. You'll also notice a difference in your skin as water reduces the appearance of wrinkles and gives the skin a healthy glow.

I don't recommend drinking water straight from the tap, however. Nearly all municipal water is routinely treated with chlorine, a potent bacteria-killing chemical, as my friend Ron Cook found out. I've installed a whole-house filtration system that removes the chlorine and other impurities from the water *before* it enters our household pipes. Nicki and I can confidently turn on the tap and enjoy the health benefits of chlorine-free water for drinking, cooking, and bathing. Since our water doesn't have a chemical aftertaste, we're more apt to drink it.

A good rule of thumb is that you should drink one quart of water for every fifty pounds of weight, so if you weigh more than 200 pounds, then you should be drinking one full gallon of water daily. I know what you're thinking: *Jordan, if I drink that much water, I can never be farther than fifteen steps from a bathroom.* Yes, you will probably treble your trips to the toilet, but trust me on this: if you're serious about controlling your blood sugar and losing weight, you must be serious about drinking enough water. There's no other physiological way for you to rid yourself of fat reserves and toxins stored inside your body.

Toxins Elsewhere in Your Environment

There are other toxins not directly related to diabetes and obesity but are important enough to mention.

Plastics

Although I occasionally drink bottled waters from plastic containers, I think it's safer to drink water from glass because dioxins and phthalates added in the manufacturing process of plastic can leach into the water, especially after reuse of the same bottle more than once.

Air Quality

We spend 90 percent of our time indoors, usually in well-insulated and energy-efficient homes and offices with central air-conditioning in the summer and forced-air heating during the winter. Double-pane windows, when tamped down shut, don't allow any fresh air into the home, and they trap "used" air filled with harmful particles such as carbon dioxide, nitrogen dioxide, and pet dander.

Perhaps you've noticed all the attention given to mold-related illnesses and homes that have been torn up to rid walls and studs of spores of green and black mold. Those living in mold-infested environments have been diagnosed with impaired thyroid and adrenal problems, chronic fatigue, and memory impairment. It's tough to stick with a lifestyle change—or remember to do so— if poor indoor air quality drains your energy.

I recommend opening your doors and windows periodically to freshen the air you breathe, even if the temperatures are blazing hot or downright freezing. Just a few minutes of fresh air will do wonders.

I also advise the purchase of a quality air filter, which will remove tiny airborne particles of dust, soot, pollen, mold, and dander. I have set up four air purifiers in our home that scrub harmful impurities out of the air.

Household Cleaners

Many of today's commercial household cleaners contain potentially harmful chemicals and solvents that expose people to VOCs—volatile organic compounds—which can cause eye, nose, and throat irritation.

Nicki and I have found that natural ingredients like vinegar, lemon juice, and baking soda are excellent substances that make our home spick-and-span. Natural cleaning products that aren't harsh, abrasive, or potentially dangerous to your family are available in natural food stores.

Skin Care and Body Care Products

Toxic chemicals such as chemical solvents and phthalates are found in lipstick, lip gloss, lip conditioner, hair coloring, hair spray, shampoo, and soap. Ladies, when you rub a tube of lipstick across your lips, your skin readily absorbs these toxins, and that's unhealthy. As with the case regarding household cleaners, you can find natural cosmetics in progressive natural food markets, although they are becoming more widely available in drugstores and beauty stores.

FINAL THOUGHT

In closing, let me be very clear that you most likely will not get sick immediately from drinking chlorinated water, breathing in recirculated air, using commercial household cleaners, rubbing chemical-laden shampoo in your hair, or even brushing your teeth with artificially flavored toothpaste, but the consistent use of these products can erode good health. By the time you notice symptoms, the damage may have already been done.

℞ THE GREAT PHYSICIAN'S Rx FOR DIABETES: REDUCE TOXINS IN YOUR ENVIRONMENT

- *Drink the minimum recommended amount of eight glasses of water daily.*

- *Use glass containers instead of plastic containers whenever possible.*

- *Improve indoor air quality by opening windows and buying an air filtration system.*

- *Use natural cleaning products for your home.*

- *Use natural products for skin care, body care, hair care, cosmetics, and toothpaste.*

- *Don't smoke cigarettes or use tobacco products.*

Take Action

To learn how to incorporate the principles of reducing toxins in your environment into your daily regimen, please turn to page 73 for the Great Physician's Rx for Diabetes Battle Plan.

KEY #6

Avoid Deadly Emotions

Did you know that anger, acrimony, apprehension, agitation, anxiety, and alarm are deadly emotions, and when you experience any of these feelings—whether justified or not—the efficiency of your immune system decreases noticeably for six hours? (This is the same amount of time your immune system shuts down when you eat large amounts of sugar.)

In addition, depression, stress, and worry may increase the risk of developing type 2 diabetes, according to a recent medical study published in *Diabetes Care*.[1] I believe negative emotions can adversely affect your health and produce lethal toxins that threaten body and spirit. My friend Don Colbert, M.D., author of the fine book *Deadly Emotions* (Thomas Nelson, 2003), says that an emotional roller coaster saps a person of both physical and psychological health, which often leaves body and mind depleted of energy and strength. Dr. Colbert points out that medical studies dealing with unhealthy emotions show that

- the mind and the body are linked, which means how you feel emotionally can determine how you feel physically.

- certain emotions release hormones into the body that can trigger the development of a host of diseases.

- researchers have directly and scientifically linked deadly emotions to hypertension, cardiovascular disease, and diseases related to the immune system.

- those fighting depression have an increased risk of developing cancer, heart disease, and diabetes, as mentioned earlier.

Deadly emotions alter the chemistry of your body, and unchecked emotions can be a pervasive force in determining your daily behavior. Eating while under stress causes the liver's bile tubes to narrow, which blocks bile from reaching the small intestine, where food is waiting to be digested. This is not healthy for those with diabetes. An old proverb states it well: "What you are eating is not nearly as important as what's eating you."

That's wise advice, but it's been my experience that when stress overwhelms people's lives, they tend to fall off the healthy food wagon. When life overwhelms them, they revert to old habits: nibbling on sweets or oily chips, raiding the refrigerator, or ordering in. They hunt down extremely pleasurable foods filled with fat and sugar—Belgian chocolates or Ben & Jerry's Cherry Garcia Ice Cream—to dampen stress and ameliorate symptoms of depression. They eat all the wrong foods to take their minds off their troubles.

These deadly emotions can produce toxins similar to a diabetic bingeing on a dozen glazed doughnuts. Those who are obese often have difficulty forgiving those who teased them about their body shape, made snide comments about their plus-size clothes, or told them that they'll never lose weight.

If you've been hurt in the past by mean-spirited comments, I'm sure I'm not the first person to urge you to put the past in the rearview mirror and move forward. But you must. If you follow my principles for a healthy lifestyle, I'm confident that this will help you deal with any deadly emotions. Please remember that no matter how bad you've been hurt in the past, it's still possible to forgive. "If you forgive men their trespasses, your heavenly Father will also forgive you," Jesus said in Matthew 6. "But if you do not forgive men their trespasses, neither will your Father forgive your trespasses" (vv. 14–15).

Give those who tormented you your forgiveness, and then let it go.

Rx THE GREAT PHYSICIAN'S Rx FOR DIABETES: AVOID DEADLY EMOTIONS

- *Don't eat when you're sad, scared, or stressed by everyday life.*

- *Recognize the interaction between having deadly emotions and having diabetes.*

- *Trust God when you face circumstances that cause you to worry or become anxious.*

- *Practice forgiveness every day and forgive those who hurt you.*

Take Action

To learn how to incorporate the principles of avoiding deadly emotions into your daily regimen, please turn to page 73 for the Great Physician's Rx for Diabetes Battle Plan.

KEY #7

Live a Life of Prayer and Purpose

Prayer is the foundation of a healthy life, linking your body, soul, and spirit to God. Prayer is a two-way communication with our Creator, the God of the universe. There's power in prayer: "The prayer of faith will save the sick" (James 5:15).

Prayer is the way we talk to God. There is no greater source of power than talking to the One who made us. Prayer is not a formality. Prayer is not about religion. Prayer is about a relationship—the hotline to heaven. We can talk to God anytime, anywhere, for any reason. He is always there to listen, and He always has our best interests at heart because we are His children.

If you decide to adopt the principles behind *The Great Physician's Rx for Diabetes* for your life, I urge you to undergird your effort with prayer, which will give you the perseverance to prevail against this disease. Seal all that you do with the power of prayer, and watch your life become more than you ever thought possible.

I'm not guaranteeing that you will experience a miraculous cure or that astonishing things will happen to you, although they often do. But I will tell you that if you treat your body as God meant for you to treat it—like a temple of the Holy Spirit (1 Cor. 6:19–20)—God will honor that.

You know, heavyset people with diabetes often ask me if overeating is a sin. While the Bible has little direct criticism of gluttony, the book of Proverbs describes the social and economic disadvantages of gluttony, which is defined as excess in eating and drinking: "Do not mix with winebibbers, or with gluttonous eaters of meat; for the drunkard and the glutton will come to poverty, and drowsiness will clothe a man with rags," says Proverbs 23:20–21.

Here's where I come down on the topic. If you're wondering whether you can overeat and not deal with the root causes of your diabetes and still get to heaven, my response is yes, you'll get to heaven. You'll just get there a lot sooner.

When you follow God's health plan, however, you'll honor your family, and the best way to honor them is by staying here on earth. I always cringe when I hear about someone involved in ministry—the pastorate, the mission field, vacation Bible school— who dies way too early because he or she did not take care of his or her body. That's a waste of God's resources here on earth.

God has a purpose for your life, and when you're called to serve Him in ministry, as I believe all of us are, every minute is precious. Every year we have more to offer, not less, because we have wisdom and experience on our side. Use that wisdom by establishing a health legacy for your future generations, and you won't live a life of regrets.

You may be reading this and thinking, *I know my diabetes is a ticking time bomb . . . and I'm not sure what my future holds.* Well, you've been given the knowledge to do something about your disease from this day forward. My question to you is: How are you going to act upon what you've learned from *The Great Physician's Rx for Diabetes*?

It matters, you know. Both of my father's grandparents had diabetes, and my mother's grandmother, Gramma Simma, had a gangrenous leg amputated late in life, which everyone in our family assumes was caused by undiagnosed diabetes.

On my father's side, my great-grandmother, Lena, died in the late 1960s because of complications of diabetes. She was very sick in her later years, suffering several strokes because her doctors couldn't get her diabetes under control. Her husband, my great-grandfather, Jacob, was also diabetic all his life, which turned out to be a long one. He died at the age of eighty-eight, but my father, who loved his grandfather very much, says he left before his time. "Poppy," he said, "wasn't insulin dependent, but he had to take medication. The night he died, he suffered a heart attack, and a pen or something in his pajama pocket punctured his heart, and he died instantly. This tragic event happened two days after my wife's father died."

As for myself, I haven't forgotten the memory of my grandfather on my father's side, who was significantly overweight, passing away at the age of sixty-two from a heart attack. My grandfather on my mother's side was overweight as well, and he died of a heart attack at the age of sixty-five. Both of my grandfathers were gone before I turned ten years old.

You don't have to die early from complications of diabetes. Give yourself the best chance to be there for your loved ones by following the principles behind *The Great Physician's Rx for Diabetes.*

Now it's your turn to take the first step on your new road to wellness. Welcome to your new, healthy life!

Start a Small Group

It's difficult to face a health challenge alone. If you have friends or family members struggling with diabetes or other health problems, or if you know people who just want to live the healthy life God intended, ask them to join you in following the Great Physician's prescription for better health. You can learn how to become a small group leader in your community or find an existing small group in your area by visiting www.GreatPhysiciansRx.com.

R̶x THE GREAT PHYSICIAN'S Rx FOR DIABETES: LIVE A LIFE OF PRAYER AND PURPOSE

- *Pray continually.*

- *Confess God's promises upon waking and before you retire.*

- *Find God's purpose for your life and live it every day.*

- *Be an agent of change in your life. Only you can take that first step toward reversing diabetes in your life.*

Take Action

To learn how to incorporate the principles of living a life of prayer and purpose into your daily regimen, please turn to page 73 for the Great Physician's Rx for Diabetes Battle Plan.

THE GREAT PHYSICIAN'S RX
FOR DIABETES BATTLE PLAN

DAY 1

Upon Waking

Prayer: thank God because this is the day that the Lord has made. Rejoice and be glad in it. Thank Him for the breath in your lungs and the life in your body. Ask the Lord to heal your body and use your experience to benefit the lives of others. Read Matthew 6:9–13 out loud.

Purpose: ask the Lord to give you an opportunity to add significance to someone's life today. Watch for that opportunity. Ask God to use you this day for His intended purpose.

Advanced hygiene: for hands and nails, jab fingers into semisoft soap four or five times, and lather hands with soap for fifteen seconds, rubbing soap over cuticles and rinsing under water as warm as you can stand. Take another swab of semisoft soap into your hands and wash your face. Next, fill basin or sink with water as warm as you can stand, and add one to three tablespoons of table salt and one to three eye-droppers of iodine-based mineral solution. Dunk face into water and open eyes, blinking repeatedly underwater. Keep eyes open underwater for three seconds. After cleaning your eyes, put your face back in the water, and close your mouth while blowing bubbles out of your nose. Come up from the water, and immerse your face in the water once again, gently taking water into your nostrils and expelling bubbles. Come up from the water, and blow your nose into facial tissue. To cleanse the ears, use hydrogen peroxide and mineral-based ear drops, putting two or three drops into each ear and letting stand for sixty seconds. Tilt your head to expel the drops. For the teeth, apply

73

two or three drops of essential oil-based tooth drops to the toothbrush. This can be used to brush your teeth or added to existing toothpaste. After brushing your teeth, brush your tongue for fifteen seconds. (Visit www.BiblicalHealthInstitute.com and click on the GPRx Resource Guide for recommended advanced hygiene products.)

Reduce toxins: open windows for one hour today. Use natural soap and natural skin and body care products (shower gel, body creams, etc.). Use natural facial care products. Use natural tooth-paste. Use natural hair care products such as shampoo, conditioner, gel, mousse, and hairspray. (Visit www.BiblicalHealthInstitute.com and click on the GPRx Resource Guide for recommended products.)

Supplements: take one serving of a fiber/green superfood powder (mixed) or five caplets of a super green formula swallowed with twelve to sixteen ounces of water. (For recommended products, visit www.BiblicalHealthInstitute.com and click on the GPRx Resource Guide.)

Body therapy: get twenty minutes of direct sunlight sometime during the day, but be careful between the hours of 10:00 a.m. and 2:00 p.m.

Exercise: perform functional fitness exercises for five to fifteen min-utes, or spend five to fifteen minutes on a mini trampoline. Finish with five to ten minutes of deep-breathing exercises. (One to three rounds of the exercises can be found at www.GreatPhysiciansRx.com.)

Emotional health: whenever you face a circumstance, such as your health, that causes you to worry, repeat the following: "Lord, I trust You. I cast my cares upon You, and I believe that You're going to take care of [insert your current situation] and make my health and make my body strong." Confess that throughout the day whenever you think about your health condition.

Breakfast

Make a vanilla-cinnamon smoothie in a blender with the follow-ing ingredients:

one cup plain whole milk yogurt or kefir (goat's milk is best); one tablespoon organic flaxseed oil; one tablespoon organic raw honey; one-half fresh or frozen organic banana; two tablespoons goat's milk protein powder (for recommended products, visit www.BiblicalHealthInstitute.com and click on the GPRx Resource Guide); one-fourth teaspoon organic ground cinnamon; dash of vanilla extract

Supplements: take two whole food multivitamin caplets and one capsule of a whole food antioxidant/energy formula with B vitamins, folic acid, and chromium (for recommended products, visit www.BiblicalHealthInstitute.com and click on the GPRx Resource Guide).

Lunch

Before eating, drink eight ounces of water.

During lunch, drink cinnamon green chai hot tea (for recommended products, visit www.BiblicalHealthInstitute.com and click on the GPRx Resource Guide) with one teaspoon of raw honey.

large green salad with mixed greens, avocado, carrots, cucumbers, celery, tomatoes, red cabbage, red peppers, red onions, and sprouts with three hard-boiled omega-3 eggs

salad dressing: use extra virgin olive oil, apple cider vinegar or lemon juice, Celtic sea salt, herbs, and spices, or mix one tablespoon of extra virgin olive oil with one tablespoon of a healthy store-bought dressing

two ounces of applesauce with one-fourth teaspoon of organic ground cinnamon

Supplements: take two whole food multivitamin caplets and one capsule of a whole food antioxidant/energy formula with B vitamins, folic acid, and chromium.

Dinner

Before eating, drink eight ounces of water.

During dinner, drink cinnamon green chai hot tea with one teaspoon of raw honey.

baked, poached, or grilled wild-caught salmon

steamed broccoli

large green salad with mixed greens, avocado, carrots, cucumbers, celery, tomatoes, red cabbage, red onions, red peppers, and sprouts

salad dressing: use extra virgin olive oil, apple cider vinegar or lemon juice, Celtic ea salt, herbs, and spices, or mix one tablespoon of extra virgin olive oil with one tablespoon of a healthy store-bought dressing

Supplements: take two whole food multivitamin caplets and one capsule of a whole food antioxidant/energy formula with B vitamins, folic acid, and chromium and one to three teaspoons or three to nine capsules of a high omega-3 cod liver oil complex (for recommended products, visit www.BiblicalHealthInstitute.com and click on the GPRx Resource Guide).

Snacks

apple slices with raw sesame butter (tahini)

one whole food nutrition bar with beta-glucans from soluble oat fiber (for recommended products, visit www.BiblicalHealthInstitute.com and click on the GPRx Resource Guide)

Drink eight to twelve ounces of water.

Before Bed

Exercise: go for a walk outdoors or participate in a favorite sport or recreational activity.

Supplements: take one serving of a fiber/green superfood powder (mixed) or five caplets of a super green formula swallowed with twelve to sixteen ounces of water.

Body therapy: take a warm bath for fifteen minutes with eight drops of biblical essential oils added.

Advanced hygiene: repeat the advanced hygiene instructions from the morning of Day 1.

Emotional health: ask the Lord to bring to your mind someone you need to forgive. Take out a sheet of paper and write the person's name at the top. Try to remember each specific action that person did against you that brought you pain. Write down the following: "I forgive [insert person's name] for [insert the action he or she did against you]." After you fill up the paper, tear it up or burn it, and ask God to give you the strength to truly forgive that person.

Purpose: ask yourself these questions: "Did I live a life of purpose today?" "What did I do to add value to someone else's life today?" Commit to living a day of purpose tomorrow.

Prayer: thank God for this day, asking Him to give you a restoring night's rest and a fresh start tomorrow. Thank Him for His steadfast love that never ceases and His mercies that are new every morning. Read Romans 8:35, 37–39 out loud.

Sleep: go to bed by 10:30 p.m.

DAY 2

Upon Waking

Prayer: thank God because this is the day that the Lord has made. Rejoice and be glad in it. Thank Him for the breath in your lungs and the life in your body. Ask the Lord to heal your body and use your experience to benefit the lives of others. Read Psalm 91 out loud.

Purpose: ask the Lord to give you an opportunity to add significance to someone's life today. Watch for that opportunity. Ask God to use you this day for His intended purpose.

Advanced hygiene: follow the advanced hygiene recommendations from the morning of Day 1.

Reduce toxins: follow the recommendations to reduce toxins from the morning of Day 1.

Supplements: take one serving of a fiber/green superfood powder (mixed) or five caplets of a super green formula swallowed with twelve to sixteen ounces of water.

Body therapy: take a hot and cold shower. After a normal shower, alternate sixty seconds of water as hot as you can stand it, followed by sixty seconds of water as cold as you can stand it. Repeat cycle four times for a total of eight minutes, finishing with cold.

Exercise: perform functional fitness exercises for five to fifteen minutes or spend five to fifteen minutes on a mini trampoline. Finish with five to ten minutes of deep-breathing exercises. (One to three rounds of the exercises can be found at www.GreatPhysiciansRx.com.)

Emotional health: follow the emotional health recommendations from the morning of Day 1.

Breakfast

two or three eggs any style, cooked in one tablespoon of extra virgin coconut oil (for recommended products, visit www.BiblicalHealthInstitute.com and click on the GPRx Resource Guide)

one slice of cinnamon-raisin sprouted or yeast-free whole grain bread (for recommended products, visit www.BiblicalHealthInstitute.com and click on the GPRx Resource Guide) with one-fourth teaspoon cinnamon, butter, and honey

one cup of spicy black chai hot tea with one teaspoon of raw honey

Supplements: take two whole food multivitamin caplets and one capsule of a whole food antioxidant/energy formula with B vitamins, folic acid, and chromium.

Lunch

Before eating, drink eight ounces of water.

During lunch, drink spicy black chai hot tea with one teaspoon of raw honey.

large green salad with mixed greens, avocado, carrots, tomatoes, red cabbage, red onions, red peppers, and sprouts with three ounces of cold, poached, or canned wild salmon

salad dressing: use extra virgin olive oil, apple cider vinegar or lemon juice, Celtic sea salt, herbs, and spices, or mix one tablespoon of extra virgin olive oil with one tablespoon of a healthy store-bought dressing

two ounces of organic applesauce mixed with one-fourth teaspoon of organic ground cinnamon

Supplements: take two whole food multivitamin caplets and one capsule of a whole food antioxidant/energy formula with B vitamins, folic acid, and chromium.

Dinner

Before eating, drink eight ounces of water.

During dinner, drink spicy black chai hot tea with one teaspoon of raw honey.

roasted organic chicken

cooked vegetables (carrots, onions, or peas, etc.)

large green salad with mixed greens, avocado, carrots, tomatoes, red cabbage, red onions, red peppers, and sprouts salad dressing: use extra virgin olive oil, apple cider vinegar or lemon juice, Celtic sea salt, herbs, and spices, or mix one tablespoon of extra virgin olive oil with one tablespoon of a healthy store-bought dressing

Supplements: take two whole food multivitamin caplets and one capsule of a whole food antioxidant/energy formula with B vitamins, folic acid, and chromium and one to three teaspoons or three to nine capsules of a high omega-3 cod-liver oil complex.

Snacks

three ounces of cottage cheese mixed with one tablespoon of flaxseed oil, one teaspoon of organic raw honey, and one-fourth teaspoon of organic ground cinnamon

one whole food nutrition bar with beta-glucans from soluble oat fiber

Drink eight to twelve ounces of water, or hot or iced fresh-brewed tea with honey.

Before Bed

Exercise: go for a walk outdoors or participate in a favorite sport or recreational activity.

Supplements: take one serving of a fiber/green superfood powder (mixed) or five caplets of a super green formula swallowed with twelve to sixteen ounces of water.

Advanced hygiene: repeat the advanced hygiene instructions from the morning of Day 1.

Emotional health: repeat the emotional health recommendations from the evening of Day 1.

Purpose: ask yourself these questions: "Did I live a life of purpose today?" "What did I do to add value to someone else's life today?" Commit to living a day of purpose tomorrow.

Prayer: thank God for this day, asking Him to give you a restoring night's rest and a fresh start tomorrow. Thank Him for His steadfast love that never ceases and His mercies there are new every morning. Read 1 Corinthians 13:4–8 out loud.

Body therapy: spend ten minutes listening to soothing music before you retire.

Sleep: go to bed by 10:30 p.m.

Day 3

Upon Waking

Prayer: thank God because this is the day that the Lord has made. Rejoice and be glad in it. Thank Him for the breath in your lungs and the life in your body. Ask the Lord to heal your body and use your experience to benefit the lives of others. Read Ephesians 6:13–18 out loud.

Purpose: ask the Lord to give you an opportunity to add significance to someone's life today. Watch for that opportunity. Ask God to use you this day for His intended purpose.

Advanced hygiene: follow the advanced hygiene recommendations from the morning of Day 1.

Reduce toxins: follow the recommendations to reduce toxins from the morning of Day 1.

Supplements: take one serving of a fiber/green superfood powder (mixed) or five caplets of a super green formula swallowed with twelve to sixteen ounces of water.

Body therapy: get twenty minutes of direct sunlight sometime during the day, but be careful between the hours of 10:00 a.m. and 2:00 p.m.

Exercise: perform functional fitness exercises for five to fifteen minutes or spend five to fifteen minutes on a mini trampoline. Finish with five to ten minutes of deep-breathing exercises. (One to three rounds of the exercises can be found at www.GreatPhysiciansRx.com.)

Emotional health: follow the emotional health recommendations from the morning of Day 1.

Breakfast

four to eight ounces of organic whole milk yogurt or cottage cheese with fruit (pineapple, peaches, or berries), honey, one-fourth teaspoon of organic ground cinnamon, and a dash of vanilla extract

handful of raw almonds

one cup of cinnamon green chai hot tea with one teaspoon of raw honey

Supplements: take two whole food multivitamin caplets and one capsule of a whole food antioxidant/energy formula with B vitamins, folic acid, and chromium.

Lunch

Before eating, drink eight ounces of water.

During lunch, drink cinnamon green chai hot tea with one teaspoon of raw honey.

large green salad with mixed greens, avocado, carrots, cucumbers, celery, tomatoes, red cabbage, red peppers, red onions, and sprouts with two ounces of low mercury, high omega-3 canned tuna (for recommended products, visit www.BiblicalHealthInstitute.com and click on the GPRx Resource Guide)

salad dressing: use extra virgin olive oil, apple cider vinegar or lemon juice, Celtic sea salt, herbs, and spices, or mix one tablespoon of extra virgin olive oil with one tablespoon of a healthy store-bought dressing

one piece of fruit in season

Supplements: take two whole food multivitamin caplets and one capsule of a whole food antioxidant/energy formula with B vitamins, folic acid, and chromium.

Dinner

Before eating, drink eight ounces of water.

During dinner, drink cinnamon green chai hot tea with one teaspoon of raw honey.

red meat steak (beef, buffalo, or venison)

steamed broccoli

baked sweet potato with butter

large green salad with mixed greens, avocado, carrots, cucumbers, celery, tomatoes, red cabbage, red peppers, red onions, and sprouts

salad dressing: use extra virgin olive oil, apple cider vinegar or lemon juice, Celtic sea salt, herbs, and spices, or mix one tablespoon of extra virgin olive oil with one tablespoon of a healthy store-bought dressing

Supplements: take two whole food multivitamin caplets and one capsule of a whole food antioxidant/energy formula with B vitamins, folic acid, and chromium and one to three teaspoons or three to nine capsules of a high omega-3 cod-liver oil complex.

Snacks

four ounces of cottage cheese or whole milk yogurt with one-fourth teaspoon organic ground cinnamon, organic raw honey, and a few almonds and raisins

one whole food nutrition bar with beta-glucans from soluble oat fiber

Drink eight to twelve ounces of water, or hot or iced fresh-brewed tea with honey.

Before Bed

Exercise: go for a walk outdoors or participate in a favorite sport or recreational activity.

Supplements: take one serving of a fiber/green superfood powder (mixed) or five caplets of a super green formula swallowed with twelve to sixteen ounces of water.

Body therapy: take a warm bath for fifteen minutes with eight drops of biblical essential oils added.

Advanced hygiene: follow the advanced hygiene instructions from the morning of Day 1.

Emotional health: follow the forgiveness recommendations from the evening of Day 1.

Purpose: ask yourself these questions: "Did I live a life of purpose today?" "What did I do to add value to someone else's life today?" Commit to living a day of purpose tomorrow.

Prayer: thank God for this day, asking Him to give you a restoring night's rest and a fresh start tomorrow. Thank Him for His steadfast love that never ceases and His mercies that are new every morning. Read Philippians 4:4–8, 11–13, 19 out loud.

Sleep: go to bed by 10:30 p.m.

DAY 4

Upon Waking

Prayer: thank God because this is the day that the Lord has made. Rejoice and be glad in it. Thank Him for the breath in your lungs and the life in your body. Read Matthew 6:9–13 out loud.

Purpose: ask the Lord to give you an opportunity to add significance to someone's life today. Watch for that opportunity. Ask God to use you this day for His intended purpose.

Advanced hygiene: follow the advanced hygiene recommendations from the morning of Day 1.

Reduce toxins: follow the recommendations for reducing toxins from the morning of Day 1.

Supplements: take one serving of a fiber/green superfood powder (mixed) or five caplets of a super green formula swallowed with twelve to sixteen ounces of water.

Exercise: perform functional fitness exercises for five to fifteen minutes or spend five to fifteen minutes on a mini trampoline. Finish with five to ten minutes of deep-breathing exercises. (One to three rounds of the exercises can be found at www.GreatPhysiciansRx.com.)

Body therapy: take a hot and cold shower. After a normal shower, alternate sixty seconds of water as hot as you can stand it, followed by sixty seconds of water as cold as you can stand it. Repeat cycle four times for a total of eight minutes, finishing with cold.

Emotional health: follow the emotional health recommendations from the morning of Day 1.

Breakfast

three soft-boiled or poached eggs

four ounces of sprouted whole grain cereal with two ounces of whole milk yogurt, one-fourth teaspoon organic ground cinnamon, almonds, and raisins (for recommended products, visit www.BiblicalHealthInstitute.com and click on the GPRx Resource Guide)

one cup of spicy black chai hot tea with one teaspoon of raw honey

Supplements: take two whole food multivitamin caplets and one capsule of a whole food antioxidant/energy formula with B vitamins, folic acid, and chromium.

Lunch

Before eating, drink eight ounces of water.

During lunch, drink spicy black chai hot tea with one teaspoon of raw honey.

large green salad with mixed greens, avocado, carrots, cucumbers, celery, tomatoes, red cabbage, red peppers, red onions, and sprouts with two ounces of low mercury, high omega-3 canned tuna

salad dressing: use extra virgin olive oil, apple cider vinegar or lemon juice, Celtic sea salt, herbs, and spices, or mix one tablespoon of extra virgin olive oil with one tablespoon of a healthy store-bought dressing

two ounces of organic applesauce with one-fourth teaspoon of organic ground cinnamon

Supplements: take two whole food multivitamin caplets and one capsule of a whole food antioxidant/energy formula with B vitamins, folic acid, and chromium.

Dinner

Before eating, drink eight ounces of water.

During dinner, drink spicy black chai hot tea with one teaspoon of raw honey.

grilled chicken breast

steamed veggies

small portion of cooked whole grain (quinoa, amaranth, millet, or brown rice) cooked with one tablespoon of extra virgin coconut oil

large green salad with mixed greens, avocado, carrots, cucumbers, celery, tomatoes, red cabbage, red peppers, red onions, and sprouts

salad dressing: use extra virgin olive oil, apple cider vinegar or lemon juice, Celtic sea salt, herbs, and spices, or mix one tablespoon of extra virgin olive oil with one tablespoon of a healthy store-bought dressing

Supplements: take two whole food multivitamin caplets and one capsule of a whole food antioxidant/energy formula with B vitamins, folic acid, and chromium and one to three teaspoons or three to nine capsules of a high omega-3 cod-liver oil complex.

Snacks

apple and carrots with raw almond butter

one whole food nutrition bar with beta-glucans from soluble oat fiber

Drink eight to twelve ounces of water, or hot or iced fresh-brewed tea with honey.

Before Bed

Drink eight to twelve ounces of water or hot tea with honey.

Exercise: go for a walk outdoors or participate in a favorite sport or recreational activity.

Supplements: take one serving of a fiber/green superfood powder (mixed) or five caplets of a super green formula swallowed with twelve to sixteen ounces of water.

Advanced hygiene: follow the advanced hygiene recommendations from the morning of Day 1.

Emotional health: follow the forgiveness recommendations from the evening of Day 1.

Purpose: ask yourself these questions: "Did I live a life of purpose today?" "What did I do to add value to someone else's life today?" Commit to living a day of purpose tomorrow.

Prayer: thank God for this day, asking Him to give you a restoring night's rest and a fresh start tomorrow. Thank Him for His steadfast love that never ceases and His mercies that are new every morning. Read Romans 8:35, 37–39 out loud.

Body therapy: spend ten minutes listening to soothing music before you retire.

Sleep: go to bed by 10:30 p.m.

DAY 5

Upon Waking

Prayer: thank God because this is the day that the Lord has made. Rejoice and be glad in it. Thank Him for the breath in your lungs and the life in your body. Read Psalm 1 out loud.

Purpose: ask the Lord to give you an opportunity to add significance to someone's life today. Watch for that opportunity. Ask God to use you this day for His intended purpose.

Advanced hygiene: follow the advanced hygiene recommendations from the morning of Day 1.

Reduce toxins: follow the recommendations for reducing toxins from the morning of Day 1.

Supplements: take one serving of a fiber/green superfood powder (mixed) or five caplets of a super green formula swallowed with twelve to sixteen ounces of water.

Exercise: perform functional fitness exercises for five to fifteen minutes or spend five to fifteen minutes on a mini trampoline. Finish with five to ten minutes of deep-breathing exercises.

Body therapy: get twenty minutes of direct sunlight sometime during the day, but be careful between the hours of 10:00 a.m. and 2:00 p.m.

Emotional health: follow the emotional health recommendations from the morning of Day 1.

Breakfast

three fried eggs in one teaspoon of extra virgin coconut oil

one serving of slow-cooked organic oatmeal with one-fourth teaspoon of cinnamon, butter, honey, and raisins

one cup of cinnamon green chai hot tea with one teaspoon of raw honey

Supplements: take two whole food multivitamin caplets and one capsule of a whole food antioxidant/energy formula with B vitamins, folic acid, and chromium.

Lunch

Before eating, drink eight ounces of water.

turkey sandwich on sprouted or yeast-free whole grain bread with natural mayonnaise, mustard, raw cheese, lettuce, and tomato

two ounces of organic applesauce with one-fourth teaspoon of organic ground cinnamon

During lunch, drink cinnamon green chai hot tea with one teaspoon of raw honey.

Supplements: take two whole food multivitamin caplets and one capsule of a whole food antioxidant/energy formula with B vitamins, folic acid, and chromium.

Dinner

Before eating, drink eight ounces of water.

During dinner, drink cinnamon green chai hot tea with one teaspoon of raw honey.

Chicken Soup (visit www.GreatPhysiciansRx.com for recipe)

cultured vegetables (for recommended products, visit www.BiblicalHealthInstitute.com and click on the GPRx Resource Guide)

large green salad with mixed greens, avocado, carrots, cucumbers, celery, tomatoes, red cabbage, red peppers, red onions, and sprouts

salad dressing: use extra virgin olive oil, apple cider vinegar or lemon juice, Celtic sea salt, herbs, and spices, or mix one tablespoon of extra virgin olive oil with one tablespoon of a healthy store-bought dressing

Supplements: take two whole food multivitamin caplets and one capsule of a whole food antioxidant/energy formula with B vitamins, folic acid, and chromium and one to three teaspoons or three to nine capsules of a high omega-3 cod-liver oil complex.

Snacks

One whole food nutrition bar with beta-glucans from soluble oat fiber

one-half cup of blueberries and a handful of almonds

Drink eight to twelve ounces of water.

Before Bed

Drink eight to twelve ounces of water or hot tea with honey.

Exercise: go for a walk outdoors or participate in a favorite sport or recreational activity.

Supplements: take one serving of a fiber/green superfood powder (mixed) or five caplets of a super green formula swallowed with twelve to sixteen ounces of water.

Advanced hygiene: follow the advanced hygiene recommendations from the morning of Day 1.

Emotional health: follow the forgiveness recommendations from the evening of Day 1.

Body therapy: take a warm bath for fifteen minutes with eight drops of biblical essential oils added.

Purpose: ask yourself these questions: "Did I live a life of purpose today?" "What did I do to add value to someone else's life today?" Commit to living a day of purpose tomorrow.

Prayer: thank God for this day, asking Him to give you a restoring night's rest and a fresh start tomorrow. Thank Him for His steadfast love that never ceases and His mercies that are new every morning. Read Matthew 6:25–34 out loud.

Sleep: go to bed by 10:30 p.m.

DAY 6 (REST DAY)

Upon Waking

Prayer: thank God because this is the day that the Lord has made. Rejoice and be glad in it. Thank Him for the breath in your lungs and the life in your body. Read Psalm 23 out loud.

Purpose: ask the Lord to give you an opportunity to add significance to someone's life today. Watch for that opportunity. Ask God to use you this day for His intended purpose.

Advanced hygiene: follow the advanced hygiene recommendations from the morning of Day 1.

Reduce toxins: follow the recommendations for reducing toxins from the morning of Day 1.

Supplements: take one serving of a fiber/green superfood powder (mixed) or five caplets of a super green formula swallowed with twelve to sixteen ounces of water.

Exercise: do no formal exercise since it's a rest day.

Body therapies: do none since it's a rest day.

Emotional health: follow the emotional health recommendations from the morning of Day 1.

Breakfast

two or three eggs cooked any style in one teaspoon of extra virgin coconut oil

one grapefruit

handful of almonds

one cup of cinnamon green chai hot tea with one teaspoon of raw honey

Supplements: take two whole food multivitamin caplets and one capsule of a whole food antioxidant/energy formula with B vitamins, folic acid, and chromium.

Lunch

Before eating, drink eight ounces of water.

During lunch, drink cinnamon green chai hot tea with one teaspoon of raw honey.

large green salad with mixed greens, avocado, carrots, cucumbers, celery, tomatoes, red cabbage, red peppers, red onions, and sprouts with three hard-boiled omega-3 eggs

salad dressing: use extra virgin olive oil, apple cider vinegar or lemon juice, Celtic sea salt, herbs, and spices, or mix one tablespoon of extra virgin olive oil with one tablespoon of a healthy store-bought dressing

two ounces of organic applesauce with one-fourth teaspoon organic ground cinnamon

Supplements: take two whole food multivitamin caplets and one capsule of a whole food antioxidant/energy formula with B vitamins, folic acid, and chromium.

Dinner

Before eating, drink eight ounces of water.

During dinner, drink cinnamon green chai hot tea with one teaspoon of raw honey.

roasted organic chicken

cooked vegetables (carrots, onions, peas, etc.)

large green salad with mixed greens, carrots, cucumbers, celery, tomatoes, red cabbage, red peppers, red onions, and sprouts

salad dressing: use extra virgin olive oil, apple cider vinegar or lemon juice, Celtic sea salt, herbs, and spices, or mix one tablespoon of extra virgin olive oil with one tablespoon of a healthy store-bought dressing

Supplements: take two whole food multivitamin caplets and one capsule of a whole food antioxidant/energy formula with B vitamins, folic acid, and chromium and one to three teaspoons or three to nine capsules of a high omega-3 cod-liver oil complex.

Snacks

handful of raw almonds with apple wedges

one whole food nutrition bar with beta-glucans from soluble oat fiber

Drink eight to twelve ounces of water, or hot or iced fresh-brewed tea with honey.

Before Bed

Drink eight to twelve ounces of water or hot tea with honey.

Exercise: go for a walk outdoors or participate in a favorite sport or recreational activity.

Supplements: take one serving of a fiber/green superfood powder (mixed) or five caplets of a super green formula swallowed with twelve to sixteen ounces of high-alkaline water or raw vegetable juice.

Advanced hygiene: follow the advanced hygiene recommendations from the morning of Day 1.

Emotional health: follow the forgiveness recommendations from the evening of Day 1.

Purpose: ask yourself these questions: "Did I live a life of purpose today?" "What did I do to add value to someone else's life today?" Commit to living a day of purpose tomorrow.

Prayer: thank God for this day, asking Him to give you a restoring night's rest and a fresh start tomorrow. Thank Him for His steadfast love that never ceases and His mercies that are new every morning. Read Psalm 23 out loud.

Body therapy: spend ten minutes listening to soothing music before you retire.

Sleep: go to bed by 10:30 p.m.

DAY 7

Upon Waking

Prayer: thank God because this is the day that the Lord has made. Rejoice and be glad in it. Thank Him for the breath in your lungs and the life in your body. Read Psalm 91 out loud.

Purpose: ask the Lord to give you an opportunity to add significance to someone's life today. Watch for that opportunity. Ask God to use you this day for His intended purpose.

Advanced hygiene: follow the advanced hygiene recommendations from the morning of Day 1.

Reduce toxins: follow the recommendations for reducing toxins from the morning of Day 1.

Supplements: take one serving of a fiber/green superfood powder (mixed) or five caplets of a super green formula swallowed with twelve to sixteen ounces of water.

Exercise: perform functional fitness exercises for five to fifteen minutes or spend five to fifteen minutes on a mini trampoline. Finish with five to ten minutes of deep-breathing exercises.

Body therapy: get twenty minutes of direct sunlight sometime during the day, but be careful between the hours of 10:00 a.m. and 2:00 p.m.

Emotional health: follow the emotional health recommendations from the morning of Day 1.

Breakfast

Make a vanilla-cinnamon smoothie in a blender with the following ingredients:

one cup plain whole milk yogurt or kefir (goat's milk is best)

one tablespoon organic flaxseed oil

one tablespoon organic raw honey

one-half fresh or frozen organic banana

two tablespoons goat's milk protein powder (for recommendations, visit www.BiblicalHealthInstitute.com and click on the GPRx Resource Guide)

one-fourth teaspoon organic ground cinnamon

dash of vanilla extract

Supplements: take two whole food multivitamin caplets and one capsule of a whole food antioxidant/energy formula with B vitamins, folic acid, and chromium.

Lunch

Before eating, drink eight ounces of water.

During lunch, drink cinnamon green chai hot tea with raw honey.

large green salad with mixed greens, raw goat cheese, avocado, carrots, cucumbers, celery, tomatoes, red cabbage, red peppers, red onions, and sprouts with three ounces of cold, poached, or canned wild-caught salmon

salad dressing: use extra virgin olive oil, apple cider vinegar or lemon juice, Celtic sea salt, herbs, and spices, or mix one tablespoon of extra virgin olive oil with one tablespoon of a healthy store-bought dressing

one piece of fruit in season

Supplements: take two whole food multivitamin caplets and one capsule of a whole food antioxidant/energy formula with B vitamins, folic acid, and chromium.

Dinner

Before eating, drink eight ounces of water.

During dinner, drink cinnamon green chai hot tea with raw honey.

baked or grilled fish of your choice

steamed broccoli

baked sweet potato with butter

large green salad with mixed greens, carrots, cucumbers, celery, tomatoes, red cabbage, red peppers, red onions, and sprouts

salad dressing: use extra virgin olive oil, apple cider vinegar or lemon juice, Celtic sea salt, herbs, and spices, or mix one tablespoon of extra virgin olive oil with one tablespoon of a healthy store-bought dressing

Supplements: take two whole food multivitamin caplets and one capsule of a whole food antioxidant/energy formula with B vitamins, folic acid, and chromium and one to three teaspoons or three to nine capsules of a high omega-3 cod-liver oil complex.

Snacks

apple slices with raw sesame butter (tahini)

one whole food nutrition bar with beta-glucans from soluble oat fiber

Drink eight to twelve ounces of water, or hot or iced fresh-brewed tea with honey.

Before Bed

Drink eight to twelve ounces of water or hot tea with honey.

Exercise: go for a walk outdoors or participate in a favorite sport or recreational activity.

Supplements: take one serving of a fiber/green superfood powder (mixed) or five caplets of a super green formula swallowed with twelve to sixteen ounces of high-alkaline water or raw vegetable juice.

Advanced hygiene: follow the advanced hygiene recommendations from the morning of Day 1.

Emotional health: follow the forgiveness recommendations from the evening of Day 1.

Body therapy: take a warm bath for fifteen minutes with eight drops of biblical essential oils added.

Purpose: ask yourself these questions: "Did I live a life of purpose today?" "What did I do to add value to someone else's life today?" Commit to living a day of purpose tomorrow.

Prayer: thank God for this day, asking Him to give you a restoring night's rest and a fresh start tomorrow. Thank Him for His steadfast love that never ceases and His mercies that are new every morning. Read 1 Corinthians 13:4–8 out loud.

Sleep: go to bed by 10:30 p.m.

DAY 8 AND BEYOND

If you are beginning to get better control of your blood sugar and feel better, but still have a way to go on your road to wellness, you can repeat the Great Physician's Rx for Diabetes Battle Plan as many times as you'd like. For detailed step-by-step suggestions and meal and lifestyle plans, visit www.GreatPhysiciansRx.com and join the 40-Day Health Experience (if you want to continue on a strict phase of the health plan) or the Lifetime of Wellness plan (if you want to maintain your newfound level of health). These online programs will provide you with customized daily meal and exercise plans and provide you with tools to track your progress.

If you've experienced positive results from the Great Physician's Rx for Diabetes program, I encourage you to reach out to others you know and recommend this book and program to them. You can learn how to lead a small group at your church or home by visiting www.GreatPhysiciansRx.com.

Remember: You don't have to be a doctor or a health expert to help transform the life of someone you care about—you just have to be willing.

Allow me to offer this prayer of blessing from Numbers 6:24–26 for you:

> May the LORD bless you and keep you.
> May the LORD make His face to shine upon you and be gracious unto you.
> May the LORD lift up His countenance upon you and bring you peace.
> In the name of Yeshua Ha Mashiach, Jesus our Messiah.
> Amen.

Need Recipes?

For a detailed list of more than two hundred healthy and delicious recipes contained in the Great Physician's Rx eating plan, please visit www.GreatPhysiciansRx.com.

NOTES

Introduction

1. Jeffrey Krasner, "Diabetes Therapy Deal," *Boston Globe,* 16 March 2005.

Key #1

1. Lyle MacWilliam, "Diabetes: Understanding and Preventing the Next Health Care Epidemic," *LifeExtension,* June 2004.

2. "Consumer Group Wants Health Warnings on Soft Drinks," ConsumerAffairs.com, July 14, 2005.

3. Associated Press, "Study: Soda May Increase Diabetes Risk for Women," *USA Today,* June 8, 2004.

4. "The Secret Dangers of Splenda (Sucralose), an Artificial Sweetener," mercola.com, http://www.mercola.com/2000/dec/3/sucralose_dangers.htm#.

5. F. Batmanghelidj, M.D., *You're Not Sick, You're Thirsty!* (New York: Warner Books, 2003), 225–26.

6. Dr. Isadore Rosenfield, "Big News About a Little Spice," *Parade,* June 13, 2004.

Key #2

1. T. A. Barringer, J. K. Kirk, A. C. Santaniello, *et al.,* "Effect of a Multivitamin and Mineral Supplement on Infection and Quality of Life," *Annals of Internal Medicine,* March 3, 2003, 365–71.

2. "Fish Oil Lowers Triglycerides with Little or No Glycemic Effect in Type 2 Diabetics," *Reuters Health,* October 2005, http://www.diabeteslibrary.org/news/news_item.cfm?NewsID=229.

Key #3

1. "Diabetes Forum," manned by the staff at Gopi Memorial Hospital in Salem Tamilnadu, India, http://www.diabetesforum.net/eng_treatment_personalHygiene.htm.

Key #4

1. Randy Dotinga, "Too Little Sleep Could Cause Diabetes," *HealthDay,* April 27, 2005, http://health.yahoo.com/news/61350.

2. Nanci Hellmich, "Sleep Loss May Equal Weight Gain," *USA Today,* December 6, 2004, http://www.usatoday.com/news/health/2004-12-06-sleep-weight-gain_x.htm.

Key #5

1. Don Colbert, M.D., *Toxic Relief* (Lake Mary, FL: Siloam, 2003), 15.

2. F. Batmanghelidj, M.D., *You're Not Sick, You're Thirsty!* (New York: Warner, 2003), 2–3.

Key #6

1. Laurent C. Brown, BSCPHARM, Sumit R. Majumdar, MD, MPH, FRCPC, Stephen C. Newman, MD, MA, MSC, and Jeffrey A. Johnson, PHD, "History of Depression Increases Risk of Type 2 Diabetes in Younger Adults," *Diabetes Care* 28:1063–1067, 2005.

ABOUT THE AUTHORS

Jordan Rubin has dedicated his life to transforming the health of others one life at a time. He is a certified nutritional consultant, a certified personal fitness instructor, a certified nutrition specialist, and a member of the National Academy of Sports Medicine.

Mr. Rubin is the founder and chairman of Garden of Life, Inc., a health and wellness company based in West Palm Beach, Florida, that produces whole food nutritional supplements and personal care products. He is also president and CEO of GPRx, Inc., a biblically based health and wellness company providing educational resources, small group curriculum, functional foods, nutritional supplements, and wellness services.

He and his wife, Nicki, married in 1999 and are the parents of a toddler-aged son, Joshua. They make their home in Palm Beach Gardens, Florida.

Joseph D. Brasco, M.D., who is board certified in internal medicine and gastroenterology, is in private practice in Indianapolis, Indiana. He has skillfully combined diet, supplementation, and judicious use of medications to provide a comprehensive and effective treatment program. Dr. Brasco is the coauthor of *Restoring Your Digestive Health* with Jordan Rubin.

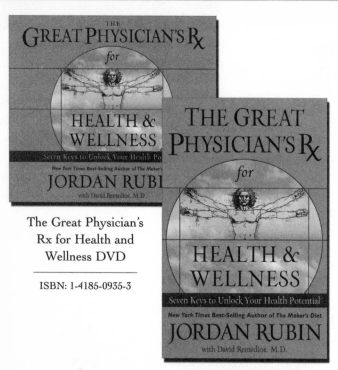

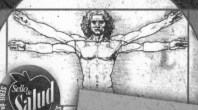
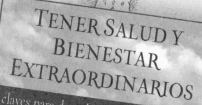

BHI

BIBLICAL HEALTH
INSTITUTE

The Biblical Health Institute (www.BiblicalHealthInstitute.com) is an online learning community housing educational resources and curricula reinforcing and expanding on Jordan Rubin's Biblical Health message.

Biblical Health Institute provides:

1. "101" level **FREE**, introductory courses corresponding to Jordan's book The Great Physician's Rx for Health and Wellness and its seven keys; Current "101" courses include:

   * "Eating to Live 101"

   * "Whole Food Nutrition Supplements 101"

   * "Advanced Hygiene 101"

   * "Exercise and Body Therapies 101"

   * "Reducing Toxins 101"

   * "Emotional Health 101"

   * "Prayer and Purpose 101"

2. **FREE** resources (healthy recipes, what to E.A.T., resource guide)

3. **FREE** media--videos and video clips of Jordan, music therapy samples, etc.--and much more!

Additionally, Biblical Health Institute also offers in-depth courses for those who want to go deeper.

Course offerings include:

   * 40-hour certificate program to become a Biblical Health Coach

   * A la carte course offerings designed for personal study and growth (launching late April 2006)

   * Home school courses developed by Christian educators, supporting home-schooled students and their parents (designed for middle school and high school ages—launching in August 2006).

**For more information and updates on these and other resources go to
www.BiblicalHealthInstitute.com**

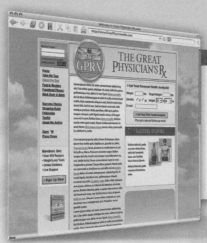

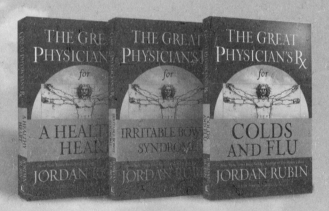

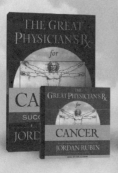
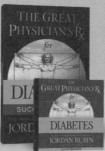
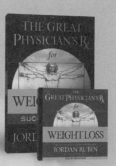